# The Fitness Lifestyle

AINSLEY BOLES LAING

ISBN: 1469920115
ISBN 13: 9781469920115

*Dedicated*
*to*
*Dave who has inspired me to write*
*and to*
*Avery who has brought joy to my life.*

# Contents

# Acknowledgments

Special thanks to my loving husband Dave who has compiled my two-year writing for the Body for Mind newsletter into The Fitness Lifestyle book.

# Foreword

Ainsley and I first began our relationship in the online world, where we spent 8 months communicating through online dating sites, video calls and text messages. Once our relationship grew into a 'real' one in 2006, we decided to move in together and share a home. During this time I was authoring a newsletter called: "Body for Mind- Wellness Lifestyle for Successful People". Ainsley began proofreading my articles and quickly became the newsletter's chief editor.

To be completely honest, at first I didn't think of Ainsley as a writer. She used pre-printed birthday cards rather than writing her own ones, so how would she be able to write uplifting, motivating and inspiring articles for my newsletter? It didn't take long for her to prove me wrong! Ainsley proved to be an amazing story-teller with plenty of passion to share.

Ainsley is a walking encyclopedia of information on fitness, nutrition, health, body, mind and self-development. She is certainly not afraid to broadcast this knowledge freely and openly whenever she can. (As it turns out she often has the opportunity to share what she knows!) At first she resisted the idea of writing about her knowledge- that was until she discovered that she could write in the same way that she spoke. This marked the beginning of her writing journey. Her ability to share her passion and knowledge helped to make our newsletter extremely success-ful because she was able to engage readers with her true life stories. Today her collection of stories offers a fantastic insight into the world of mind and body health.

Ainsley's expansive scientific background is also evident in her writing. This background is reflected in how well she writes about topics that too often are filled with hype and misinformation. In contrast, Ainsley offers meticulous research and a scientific approach to her writings regarding mind and body fitness.

For years I have had an irresistible urge to share with the world the wealth of wisdom and knowledge that Ainsley shares with me each and every day. I love to read Ainsley's stories and I hope that you will as well. She was not aware that I had been compiling her collection of stories to print, so this book will come as a surprise!

I am extremely grateful that Ainsley and I share a common passion regarding mind and body fitness. It has allowed us to share a wonderful life together. After all, Ainsley is my personal trainer, my lover, my co-parent and my wonderful wife.

*DAVE OSH 2012*

# FITNESS

# To Stretch or
# Not to Stretch...

I started teaching fitness classes a long time ago. So long ago, in fact, that Jane Fonda was THE NAME in fitness and all the classes were called Aerobics. In those days, there was no certification for instructors and most of us came from a dance background. In other words, we did what we wanted with very few guidelines.

Along with the increase in popularity of these classes and fitness in general came certification, liability insurance, expert guidelines and large amounts of scientific research on fitness topics. In other words, teaching fitness classes became a "real job".

Since that time, stretching seems to be a really controversial area of fitness. When do we stretch? How do we stretch? Does stretching prevent injury? Do you get sore if you stretch properly? And you know what? After many studies later, the mysteries remain.

Of course, there are a couple of generally accepted beliefs I would like to share with you to help you better understand and plan your fitness activities.

1.  A muscle's strength is related to its ability to stretch. In other words a muscle expands before it contracts. This is particularly easy to see when you look at someone jump. First the person will bend the knees (expand the muscles) and then spring up (contract).

2.  A warm muscle stretches more easily than a cold one. The follow on to this idea is that a warm muscle is also stronger in that it is more resistant to tearing with heavy use.

How is this applied to fitness programs? Well, the number one thing I always say to my clients is "Warm-up first before stretching". The response from clients is often, "Isn't stretching a warm-up"? The answer is (polite yet emphatic) NO!

The purpose of a warm-up is to get the blood flowing to the muscles and joints and get the heart ready for what is to come. The best warm-up is usually about 5 minutes of a lower intensity version of the activity you are about to perform. For example, walking for a time before you begin running is good. For weight training, it's also good to walk first followed by some rhythmic arm movements to warm up upper body joints.

Now here's a big controversy among fitness professionals: when is the optimal time to stretch? Well, I like to stretch at the end of the workout or at several times during the workout if resistance (weight) training – when the muscles are very bendable. My mental picture of this is that muscles, tendons and ligaments are like taffy candy. When taffy is cold, it breaks when bent. When taffy is warm, it pulls and stretches.

While no one has yet managed to prove conclusively that stretching prevents injury or reduces muscle soreness, most athletes and fitness enthusiasts will tell you that stretching really helps them feel better after a workout. My personal observation is that stretching promotes a balanced range of motion in the joints and generally promotes the feeling of relaxed well-being after a workout. Some of my most popular classes end with a stretching session and a few minutes of deep breathing/deep relaxation. Very nice!

# Is Body Awareness an Undergarment?

A while back my husband, who is a big fitness enthusiast and keeps himself in very good shape, began working out with me. Smart guy – he knows how to use the resources available to him!

Anyway, as we started working out, it became evident very quickly that even though his fitness level is quite high, he has developed some training habits that have led to muscular imbalances. Hence, this chapter...

By the way, he said it was "OK" to use his body for discussion in this chapter.

So, what is a muscular imbalance? The technical definition is: when two opposing muscle groups do not have comparable strength levels. In other words, it is when the body part or limb is stronger on one side than the other. Over time this lopsided development results in complications like poor posture and joint instability.

My husband is not the only one with imbalances. All of us have some muscular imbalances just because in our daily lives we move in certain ways over and over. Exercise can help alleviate this because the body does different motions than it's used to. However, doing the same exercises or sports the same way over and over can also lead to muscular imbalances.

Muscular imbalances can contribute to injury. Just like a team of people, when all the muscles needed to perform a task aren't working together, the other muscles and tendons "take up the slack". This makes the strong ones stronger and leaves the weaker ones weaker. As well, the joints (which include the vertebrae of the back) can be pulled out of alignment by the imbalance....

On the flip side, having an injury can lead to muscular imbalances. Last year, I seriously pulled a muscle in the back of my leg. I took some time off from fitness to let it heal and then took extra care not to overwork or injure it again. This meant changing the way I did some exercises and omitting other exercises for a while. Sometime later, my massage therapist told me that although my leg had long since healed, I was not strengthening it. I thought I had been working it hard! So, I watched myself in the mirror and noticed that I was compensating with the other leg and creating imbalance. Lesson learned.

So what to do? Become more "body aware". Check out your body and how you are moving it. Here are some ideas:

- Use a mirror to check out your movements. If you are unsure how an exercise or movement should be, a good book or video on training form is a good idea.

- Add yoga, ballet, tai chi or another activity that requires the mind to be fully focused on individual muscle movements in a slow, concise and specific fashion.

- Stretch all the muscle groups after exercise.

- Hire a trainer. A certified fitness trainer has the knowledge and skills to help you identify potential and existing imbalances in your body and prescribe exercises to prevent or correct them.

Enjoy more balance in your life!

# Too Much of a Good Thing?

We have all heard the term "overtraining", but what does the term mean really? Well, it means different things to different people depending on what activity or sport is involved. Mostly it means too much, too often and too intense.

If you have been weight/resistance training, you will understand how great it is to see your body change so dramatically and how easy it would be to increase training intensity and frequency too quickly. Of course, rationally we all know this is a mistake. But, the desire for an even better shape and "feel good" chemicals (endorphins) can cause us to do just a bit too much… ouch.

I had this experience when I started training with weights 15 years ago. I had been teaching aerobics classes for 8 years when I started. Well, naturally the weights changed my body a lot and I LIKED the changes! Then one day, I decided to do the same workout twice in one day. I mean, after all, if one is good, two is better right? Wrong! The result was tendonitis in my shoulder which took forever to heal.

Now, often I spend a fair bit of time explaining to clients how more is not necessarily better. The key is to workout SMART! Ok, what does this mean?

First: rest is very important. Muscles need rest between workouts. Working the same muscles in the same way too often results in injury and a reduction in performance. When a muscle is overtired, the load is taken into the joint. Joints are not designed for load, they are designed for movement. Tendonitis and joint pain are pretty common indicators of overtraining.

Second: varied workouts. This is why we fitness instructors recommend doing different sports or fitness activities. But for "die hard" weight lifters, variation can be accomplished in a variety of ways. One common way is to work different muscle groups in different days. Another method is to change the way in which a particular exercise is performed so as to train the muscles differently. An example of this would be to change the speed of the lift from workout to workout, like very slow one day and faster the next time the muscle group is worked.

There's lots of ways to vary your workouts. Check out some books on weight training or talk to a Fitness Trainer if you need some ideas. You will help prevent injury, and you will see changes in your strength.

Keep your workouts SMART!

# Have a Six Pack

Just yesterday, I was talking to my friend Jack, who is a Tri-athlete. To train, he runs, swims, cycles and lifts weights. I hadn't seen this guy for about 6 months and he has really changed his body quite a bit with his rigorous training schedule. He was showing me how his body had changed and asked me, "what else can I do to strengthen my abdominals?" My answer, as always, was very long winded... and inspired this chapter. Thanks Jack!

There has been a paradigm shift in the last few years in fitness science about how to strengthen abdominals. Have you heard the term core body strength? Then you have heard about this trend. What is means is that in order to strengthen the abdominals, all of the muscles of the front, side and back of the torso must be exercised. It also includes strengthening the pelvic floor muscles! This is because all of these muscles work synergistically to stabilize the middle of the body.

Using the core training philosophy will not only improve those wash board abs, but will help your posture and ability to avoid back injury. To implement this doesn't necessarily mean doing different exercises than you are already doing, so long as you are working out your abdominals, obliques and spinal erectors (lower back). It means doing them differently.

Here are 2 core techniques that will improve your workout:

1. Pull your pelvic floor muscles up (yes men too!) Women who have been pregnant will remember doing Kegel exercises. Same movement, but you want to practice holding these muscles up at all times during your workout. As your pelvic floor muscles get stronger, you will start to notice that when you pull them up, your lower abdominals tighten up. This is because of the interconnection of the muscles of the abdominal wall and the pelvic floor muscles.

2. Pull your belly button towards your spine. This motion engages all the ab muscles.

I highly recommend that you apply these 2 core techniques not only when you are doing abdominal exercises, but when you are doing ANYTHING. Using these techniques for abdominal work increases the focus of the exercise and the number of muscles worked. Using these techniques when running or weight lifting displaces the force throughout the core, which will result in better balance and stability and less downward compression on the spine.

If you would like to know more about core body work, there are tons of books and workout videos on the subject. Another really good way to learn about core work is to take a Pilates class, Stability Ball class or Bosu. This philosophy is becoming very popular and as such there are new core workouts coming out all the time. Ask your trainer or at your gym about them.

# AM or PM Workouts

Here's a question that I hear from clients in my fitness classes a lot: "Is it better to workout in the morning or evening?" My answer – "It depends".

It depends primarily on your lifestyle....what fits into your schedule easily is going to be something that you can stick with long-term. And since becoming and staying fit is really a lifestyle (after all, you gotta keep doing it!) it's best to make sure the timing works for you.

There is a lot of discussion among fitness enthusiasts about the physiology behind exercise and the times of day that people work out. Athletes and serious competitors use timing to structure their workouts and optimize their training. But, for us regular fitness buffs, it's helpful to be aware of this physiology and time of day to help us prevent injury and get the most out of our workouts.

When we sleep, our bodies are at a lower body temperature. First thing in the morning, our muscles and joints are still cold from sleep and our blood and synovial fluid (joint lubricant) is a bit viscous. You may notice how your feel a bit "stiff" when you first get out of bed. This is why.

Think of your muscles as being like taffy candy. When taffy is cold, it is hard and brittle. When it warms up, it stretches a really long way. Likewise, when your muscles are cold, they will not stretch so easily and are more likely to tear if taxed too heavily.

Think of your joints like the mechanical parts of a car engine. Engines require motor oil to function smoothly. When an engine is cold its motor oil is thicker and gooier than when the engine is warmed up. The parts of the engine run more smoothly when the oil is warm. The same is true with the synovial fluid of your joints. Cold joints move less smoothly because the fluid that lubricates them is thicker.

Now back to the muscles. A muscle's strength depends on not only its ability to contract, but also its ability to extend or stretch. This is referred to as the "tensile strength" of the muscle.  A cold muscle has a lowered tensile strength – so it's just not as strong.

So, it stands to reason that if you work out first thing in the morning, to prevent muscle injury and wear and tear of your joints, it's good to give yourself a bit longer warm up period than if you work out in the afternoon.

If you have the chance, do your work outs at different times of day and see if you are stronger in the morning or afternoon (most research tells us that people are stronger in the afternoon).  Doing this also changes your body's response to your workouts, meaning that the same workout will affect you differently at different times of day.

So, the answer to the question: "Is it best to workout in the morning or evening?"….. "It depends on when you LIKE to workout!"

# Work Hard, Relax
# and Breathe Deeply

So, you've just completed a really good heart pumping, muscle exhausting workout. You stretch briefly and into the shower. Another day's mission accomplished. But in the back of your mind, there's a nagging feeling that your workouts are missing something.

Now, if you are like me, you are overwhelmed with the "should do's" and "must do's" with regards to fitness (and I'm a fitness instructor!). Every week there's something new and the message seems to be that if we don't do it, we are not going to be the most fit we can be. What's a fitness buff to do?

Relax that's what! No I mean that literally. After an exhilarating workout, the body is hot, the muscles are stretchy and the mind is full of feel good chemicals...the perfect state for a few minutes of deep relaxation.

No time you say? Well, how about including deep breathing in your stretching routine? It adds no time to your stretch (after all you are doing it anyway, aren't you?) and really increases the oxygen to the muscles.

Over the last couple of years, since the advent of the popularity of mind/body (yoga, pilates etc.) exercise methods, I have started including some techniques into my regular classes and asked for feedback. After all, most of my clients are very busy people who want "all in one" workouts with results.

There's one popular technique that I found easy to implement that you can try. I must warn you in classes it's common for people to fall asleep doing this!

After you finish your workout and cool down (your heart rate is no longer elevated) try this:

1. Lie down on your back
2. Tell your whole body to relax and sink into the floor

3.  Breathe in very slowly while counting to 7 slowly (think: 1 and 2 and 3 and...).
4.  Breathe out slowly to the count of "7 and 6 and 5 and....to 1.
5.  Repeat the breath cycles 5 times to get the feel for it.
6.  Now begin your regular stretches using the same breathing technique.
7.  Hold each stretch for 2 or 3 breath cycles.

Take note of how the muscles relax into the stretch with each breath cycle.

Wow! There's something really nice about how the body and mind feels after stretching and deep breathing. I find that when I concentrate on my breathing and stretching, there's no room in my brain for thinking about anything else – no worries allowed...

Next time you stretch, try it. It's a great way to teach your body to relax after a workout and to really improve your flexibility...both physical and mental!

# Funny, I Don't Feel
# Like a Master Athlete!

This last weekend, I met with someone who I haven't seen for 8 years or so. This person, a quiet and very kind man, was my training partner for my first marathon 12 years ago. It was great to see him – not only because he looks so fit and healthy at age 57, but also because it was only this weekend that I truly felt the way that he "touched" my life so many years ago.

You see, training for a marathon is a long journey. So many hours and months my partner and I spent running, thinking about running, planning for running, eating for running....do you get the idea? Of course, achieving the goal was that much more sweet because of how hard the journey was. That one journey got me hooked and I have done many more since. But the first one remains the most special.

My marathon partner was 45 when he ran his FIRST marathon. He is quite an inspiration!

As a person who is "into fitness" I have many friends and colleagues who are sports people. Not only that, but most of them (me included) are now of the age that they are called Master Athletes. What is a master athlete? This is someone who competes in the older age categories of a sport.

So, most of my friends and I are masters in our sports. Among my peers, I hear a lot of moaning about how we are getting older and just don't feel able to compete with the youngsters. To that, I say…. Experience and science is starting to show otherwise.

Have you noticed that there are a lot of professional and amateur athletes that are still getting better at their sports even though they are also older than they are "supposed" to be?

There are many reasons for this phenomenon, but training methods, nutrition science and just plain old determination not to retire is fueling much of this.

The activities of these older athletes and the fact that there are so many now have some important lessons for those of us who feel that old age is a reason not to be fit and/or enjoy whatever sport we choose.

We can excel at sports or be as fit as someone much younger, so long as we keep some basic ideas in mind:

1.  The decline in fitness is very gradual as we age. In other words, there's no reason to stop JUST because of age.
2.  Recovery from intense training slows as we age, not the ability to train intensively.
3.  Muscular strength, flexibility and quickness (power) require extra attention to maintain, to keep us in the game and injury free.
4.  Eating right helps recovery.
5.  Adequate sleep is important for recovery.

Let's look at these ideas individually:

The decline in fitness is really just a de-training effect. If you don't use it, you lose it. Age has much less to do with this decline than inactivity does. When you were 20, if you didn't exercise, what happened? Probably, you got weaker and put on body fat. Is there much difference now years later?

Recovery time has to do with the body's ability to regenerate. Of course, the body adapts to the loads placed on it at any age; so if you GRADUALLY begin to train your body more often or more intensively, it will adapt to this training and "learn" to recover faster.

Muscular strength, flexibility and ability to respond quickly diminish without training.

The lack of muscular strength causes the joints to carry more of the load. When the joints carry the load instead of the muscles then the joints tend to break down in a variety of ways. So, it's important to build all the muscles of the body no matter what sport you are involved in.

The tensile strength of muscles, or their ability to stretch, lessens when they are not regularly stretched, so it's important to take extra care to stretch the muscles when they are warm. A tight muscle leads to muscular imbalances which again can cause joints and the back to carry loads in a way they were not designed to.

Joints tend to deteriorate with age. They lose the collagen matrix and "squishy stuff" that lubricates them. Keeping the muscles strong and flexible, so that they themselves do the work instead of the joints, is the best way to slow this deterioration. Also, if you already have joint pain, strengthening the muscles will lessen the load on the joint...and hence lessen any pain and stiffness.

Nutrition science has come a long way in recent years. Nowadays, athletes are using nutrition to aid in recovery. The crux of this is that eating lots of antioxidant rich foods (fruits and vegetables), protein (meat, fish, dairy, beans, eggs) and lots of water help the muscles rebuild and alleviates oxidative stress from exertion.

There are many supplements that have been proven, such as glucosamine for joint health, that can help with individual issues. So, if you are training hard and feel that your nutrition is less than optimal, it might be beneficial to consider supplements. It's a good idea to study up on anti-aging supplements and general nutrition guidelines to see what might benefit you.

The body uses sleep time to recover and build. Enough said on that.

The moral of the story? Age by itself is not a good excuse for not doing the things you love to do. If you have always dreamed of running a marathon – GO FOR IT!

# Fitness is a Gift to Others

Last week, a friend of mine was telling me about her 2 aunts. Both are about 60 years old. One aunt has always been athletic and fit and the other has always been sedentary. Now, at 60, the fit aunt is still active and the sedentary aunt is still sedentary – only she has trouble standing up from a chair!

After my friend told this story, I kept thinking about how much more fun the fit aunt must be to her family and friends than the sedentary one.

I feel that, although we think we do it for ourselves, being fit and healthy is a gift to our family, friends and the community in which we live. This is true in so many ways. Here's just a few of them.

## For our Family:

For our spouses, we give them the gift of being paired with someone who looks good and feels good. Waking up everyday next to someone who has the energy and spirit to embrace the day is life enriching.

Does the "looks good" comment sound superficial? Think about this. How does it feel to be at a social function and know that the man or woman across the room receiving "attention" from people his/her own age (or even younger) is the person that chooses to be with you everyday? It feels good doesn't it? This feeling is a gift to our spouse.

Superficialities aside, we give our spouses many other gifts by being fit. Better sex and love making is a very important one! Fit people have more strength, endurance, energy and better blood flow. All these contribute to better sex…. Not to mention feeling good about our own body helps us to be freer with our partners.

By being fit and healthy, we increase our spouse's confidence in having a long and active life with us. A wonderful gift indeed!

For our children, we give them the gift of healthy, active parents. Having fit parents is predictive of our children being fit themselves. We give them the gift of being more patient and helpful to them because we have the physical resources to do so. We give them the freedom from worry that we will require hospice care while they are still young adults raising their own kids.

For our grandkids, we give them the gift of being able to play with them - I mean really play with them. How proud will they be to have such "cool" grandparents? We show them how important fitness is to living long, active and fun lives.

For our sisters and brothers, we give them the gift of being loved by someone who respects themselves enough to take extra good care of their body.

## For Our Friends:

We give them the gift of having lots of energy for them. Cultivating good friendships on top of meeting family obligations requires energy – and being fit gives us the energy and health to "go the extra distance" with our friends at middle age and later in life.

## For Our Community:

We remain healthier longer and don't place a burden on the health system. We remain productive, enthusiastic members of the workforce longer. After retirement, we have time and energy to volunteer our services and skills for worthy causes. We help younger people see and feel that aging is not something to be afraid of. We are able to help those who need us.

## For Our world:

Every workout, every nutritious meal, every full night's sleep and every other way we take care of our bodies are gifts to someone else. It's not about being selfish. It's about keeping the body healthy so that the mind and spirit can contribute to the lives of others better and longer.

# Fairy Tale Fitness

At University, many years ago, I took a class in marketing. One of the lessons of this class was about the "Cinderella Theme" in marketing and merchandising. Have you ever heard of it? Even if you don't know it by its technical name, I am quite sure you would recognize this method or philosophy.

Guys, how many of you have wanted a car just because that particular car has the image of being a "Babe Magnet"? Be honest with yourself now – 99% of you, right? This is how the professionals on Madison Avenue make their living.

Ladies, how much make-up do you have in your make-up bag that you bought because the model looked good, the guy in the ad looked good.....only to get the cosmetic home and find it makes you feel like a clown?

Those folks on Madison Avenue are good...I personally keep buying lipsticks that when I buy them I just know this is the magic one that will change my looks and hence my life forever - only to find I look the same with different colored lips. Ah well.

After many years helping fitness clients, I feel that some clients also begin a fitness program with a "Cinderella" mentality. If I had a dollar for every time I heard someone say "If only I could lose 10 pounds, I would be so much happier", I would be pretty rich by now.

Just imagine how much money is made appealing to this thinking with quick fixes such as diet pills, weight loss suits, diet foods, etc. The list is exhausting.

It really doesn't matter with respect to fitness how or why a person decides to get fit and change their body composition – the end result is the same. What gets them to the decision, be it vanity, peer pressure, health or Madison Avenue doesn't make any difference....so long as the commitment is made.

The equation is the same: commit the time, do the work and you will lose fat, gain muscle and get fit.

But, here's where the fairy tale ends. A great many people will commit and follow through only long enough to reach a goal. I feel that this is the Cinderella theme aspect of all this. Many clients I have seen see "weight loss", or "getting into a size 7" as a goal and use fitness programs and/or diets as a means to get there. Again, a good reason to start; but just losing a few pounds does not make a fit, strong body and heart nor does the weight stay off permanently.

Slim people are not necessarily fit....fit people are not necessarily slim. I recently read some scary statistics somewhere that concluded that many women were smoking cigarettes because they believed this would keep them slim. Since smoking is counterproductive to fitness, I would guess that these slim people are not as fit as they could be! But, I digress.

Fitness takes time, is hard work and needs to continue for some time for a person to really transform into "the princess" or "prince". I generally tell clients that, although it takes about 6 months to start to feel "the magic" of getting fit by following a good fitness and nutrition plan, it takes much more time to get real, lasting changes in both body composition and health profile.

It is true that the practicalities of getting fit, staying fit and making healthy lifestyle choices don't seem romantic. They involve sweat, tears and just plain old time - a lifetime in fact.

It's about the process, small increments over a long time period. Through the process, a self-romance can grow: a sense of pride of accomplishment and a strong beautiful body. THE PROCESS is the "happily ever after"...

# Kids Don't Work Out, They Play

The other day, I was working out to music in my living room when my 8 year old daughter and two of her friends came in. Naturally, questions followed: what am I doing, why am I doing it, etc. After a while, the three of them joined in.

Of course, kids being kids, my workout soon expanded into a free movement and dance session. The sound levels increased with lots of laughter and squeals. After a while, the festive atmosphere was too attractive even for a grown up friend of mine to resist and she joined in. What started as a workout became a party!

Kids have such an amazing way of moving just to move which we adults sometimes forget how to do. With a few exceptions (obesity, physical disability etc) kids don't need organized workouts, personal trainers, posh workout clothes or equipment to get them moving. Have you ever watched children playing on a playground? Now that's a tough work out! They move, run, jump, tumble down and get up again over and over. They move because moving feels good, not because they "have to" or "need to" exercise.

Most of us adults did a fair number of physical activities involving free play when we were young. How many of those activities do we do now? If not, why not? The common phrase I hear from adults (I have heard myself say this) is "I used to be able to do that, but now I am too old".

Honestly, is being too old a valid reason or just an excuse to allow ourselves not to do something? Personally, when I say "I am too old to do that", I really mean I am afraid of hurting myself. I know I was afraid of getting hurt as a kid too. What did I say back then? Certainly not "I am too old". I would have said, I am afraid of hurting myself…then I would give it a try – again and again.

This idea of giving up things as we become "too old" seems to be a self-fulfilling prophesy. Stopping activities because we are too old means becoming more sedentary and hence less excited about daily life…just plain old. To quote Barbara Morris, author of "Put Old on Hold": Who decides when you are old? You Do!

Ok, ok, of course, many of you reading this would disagree. But more and more people are saying "I am not going to stop doing activities that I did when I was younger". Stopping is just not an option for these determined and vibrant people. Of course, because of past injuries, safety issues or whatnot, the way of doing the activities might have to be modified.

Back to the free play idea...free play is about learning. Learning keeps us young. This is true for our bodies as well as our brains. Our bodies learn with use or unlearn with disuse. If we are doing the same activity over and over, our bodies will learn to do those things very well and will unlearn those things that we don't do anymore. Likewise, our bodies will learn to do new things that we take up.

We fitness trainers convey this notion to clients as a "practical explanation" that there is a need to do a variety of activities to keep from hitting a fitness plateau and losing motivation – often referred to as cross training. It would be very difficult to convince adults that they need to go to the playground and just play like a kid, so we apply lots of science and logic to the argument. But free play is the message. New experiences, challenges and fun keep us young.

As an example, my spouse, a 40-something fitness buff, recently decided that he wanted to take up something completely new for his body, Kung Fu. After the first lesson he said that he was really sore and said he felt injured because "the guy really did hit me hard". I thought for sure he wouldn't continue. The next day he was buying special Kung Fu shoes with great enthusiasm. Hmm ...like a kid on the playground he tries, gets hurt and tries again. Why? Because he is doing it - FOR FUN.

Although, doing the same activities over and over is a comfortable routine, getting out of the comfort zone expands us physically, mentally and spiritually. How to get out of the comfort zone? Play like a kid!

# Fitness, Friends and Core Values

The other day I came across a quotation that said something like "if you want to know about a man's character, look at his friends". This statement really made me stop and think about not just how our friends influence our behavior; but how we tend to choose our friends based on our core values. These core values are reflected in the activities that we choose to engage in, which affords us the opportunity to meet people with the same interests and hopefully similar values.

If you are involved with kids and adolescents in any way, you are probably familiar with how much influence a child or teenager's peers have on their behavior. The example that comes to mind is the study that shows that a teen is much more likely to smoke cigarettes, drink alcohol or take drugs if his/her peers do so. Peer pressure is very strong for young people whose values are not yet formed or defined in a way that they become part of the person's character (behavior choices). To put it simply, kids need experience, education and guidance to learn to make the right choices for themselves.

What about adults? It has been my observation that a similar thing applies. As adults, we are expected to be responsible for our own behavior but we also crave approval from people close to us. But, for most of us our value systems are well defined which keeps us from following blindly after someone whose values we don't agree with. Most adults are not particularly comfortable around people whose behavior contradicts their own value system.

We become very concerned when our friends exhibit behavior that contradicts what we believe their values to be. An example of this would be when a recovering alcoholic starts drinking again. This person has demonstrated that he/she values his/her health but suddenly begins the activity that led to poor health to begin with. It's very disappointing to see someone we admire make poor choices for themselves, no matter what reasons they have for it.

We like our friends and family to be proud of the way we live our lives, but we also want to have friends whose life choices we are proud of. We choose "high quality" friends because we consider ourselves to be "high quality". We have expectations for ourselves and our choice of friends and partners is a reflection of those expectations.

Applying this to fitness: when you joined a gym and began a fitness and healthy eating program, what happened?

- Did you find that your well- meaning non fit friends inadvertently sabotaged your efforts with comments like, "You are already skinny why do you need to work out or diet? Come to "happy hour" with us instead". Did you feel enthusiastically supported?

- Through your new fitness activity, did you meet new people who you admired because they too made a commitment to take care of their health and have followed through? Did you feel a sense of association and belonging with this new set of fitness enthusiasts?

While it's important to keep our existing friends and family close when we decide to make life changes, it's also helpful to develop a new network friends who are role models, mentors and advocates: people who are succeeding to do what it is we are endeavoring to do. This idea is often discussed within the topic of business and management success. There are many dieting support groups out there that encourage mentoring. In fitness, personal trainers do a lot of mentoring/coaching. Many also introduce their clients to one another and form support groups or plan social activities.

Having a network of fitness friends will help you stay on track working towards your goals or, more importantly, will question you when you start getting off track. They will challenge you to take yourself to the next level.

Not only is having friends to work out with more fun, but these same people will genuinely celebrate your small victories with you – because they will know how hard you have worked to achieve them. Their appreciation for your accomplishments will feel great because you admire them for what they are doing – and you are doing it too!

# Is Exercising to Burn Fat and Exercising to Burn Calories the Same Thing?

Over the weekend, a really good friend was discussing how he "just can't seem to lose 2 kilos". He feels that it is fat weight and we discussed ways in which he can change his workout to optimize fat loss. This got me started thinking about how many different methods of fat loss and fads have come and gone over the many years that I have been a fitness instructor.

If there is one thing I have learned – exercising regularly over time will work to burn fat. The methods that work for each individual vary depending on the individual's weight, cardiovascular fitness level, activity level, metabolism, muscle development, size and even gender!

For all of us, though, if we eat more than our body requires – we either store it as fat or have to "burn it off".

The body at rest uses energy (calories) to power the organs, brain, cardiovascular system, immune system and skeletal muscle. In other words, all of the cells of the body require energy. The rate in which the body uses energy to function is known as the basal metabolic rate. There are two other areas of calorie requirements, one known as the thermic effect of eating (energy required to digest food) and the thermic effect of exercise.

So how does the body convert energy for use during exercise? There are 3 principle metabolic pathways, which are the ways in which the body produces Adenosine Triphosphate (ATP). I promise not to go too technical here and risk boring you...

1. *The ATP-PCr System*

   This is used during the first few seconds of exercise. Creatine phosphate (PCr) in the blood is used to produce ATP which powers the cells.

2. *The Glycolytic System*

Glycolysis means the breakdown of glucose. The body uses this system for the first few minutes of exercise.

If the exercise is very intense (say sprinting), glucose in the blood is used without oxygen and the byproduct of this will be lactic acid. After a while, the lactic acid accumulates (the burning sensation in the muscle) and leads to muscle failure. This is known as anaerobic or fast glycolysis.

If the exercise is less intense (jogging), glucose in the blood is used with oxygen to produce ATP and the byproduct will be pyruvate which then is used by the oxidative system below. This is known as aerobic or slow glycolysis.

3. *The Oxidative System*

This system has 4 parts which I definitely won't go into except to give you the names: slow glycolysis (discussed above), the Krebs Cycle, Electron Transport Chain and Beta Oxidation.

In this system, fats more than carbohydrates (glucose) are used to generate ATP. This process is called lipolysis. The fat produces more "energy" (ATP molecules), but also requires more oxygen.

What Does It All Mean?

In order to burn  more fat, the intensity level must be kept at a level that is sustainable for long enough to move into the "fat burning zone" or Oxidative System.

Most people have about 2 hours of stored glycogen (glucose) in the muscle when exercising at moderate intensity. So it's safe to assume that unless you are running a marathon, you are using both stored glucose and fat when doing your aerobic training. This applies to whatever type of aerobic training you choose. Weight training, on the other hand, relies on stored available carbohydrate (glucose) because the short duration/high intensity of each lift doesn't call for the body to burn fat for fuel.

The argument that low intensity long duration exercise burns a greater percentage of calories from fat still stands. Example: a comparison of the calories expended by the same person walking for 1 hour and jogging for 1 hour reveals that the walking burns a much greater percentage of calories from fat although the overall calorie expenditure is lower.

In terms of just pure calorie consumption during exercise – the more oxygen you use the greater your calorie use. If we look at the Oxidative System which uses fat, but requires more oxygen to do, we can infer that working out at medium intensity for longer durations will burn more calories AND a higher percentage of fat.

The current thinking is that the more muscle groups engaged during the activity (example: aerobic dance with arms and legs), the harder the body works requiring more oxygen and more calories. Do it long enough, the body will burn a higher percentage of fat.

There's a lot of discussion about the "afterburn" or the thermic effect of exercise recovery. Yes, the body does burn energy to recover. A more intense workout requires more energy to recover – hence more calories burned after the workout.

There are many fitness programs that advocate interval aerobics for fat burning. There are just as many that advocate long duration aerobics for fat burning. I advocate a combination of the 2. Both will burn fat. Each has benefits beyond fat burning.

Interval training increases your cardiovascular strength, output, heart rate recovery and produces a stronger "afterburn".

Long duration trains the cardiovascular system to sustain an increased load for a longer period of time and teaches the body to convert fat to energy more efficiently for use during exercise (endurance).

Whatever aerobic activity a person does, the key is to keep doing it. Why? The more a person exercises, the more efficient the body becomes at converting and using available carbohydrate and fat. So... regular aerobic exercise over a long period of time is more important for fat and calorie burning than which method used.

# Body Fitness
# Equals Brain Fitness

Have you always thought that athletes were less intelligent? Well, hold on to your hat...more and more research supports the idea that the brains of exercisers function better.

This is not new. Researchers have known for years that the brains of exercisers were more active and pliable in later life. Many recent studies take this a step further.

In one such study, Charles Hillman, a professor at the University of Illinois, noticed that over and over the women in his classes that were on the cross-country team consistently scored higher on his exams. Hillman wondered about the possible fitness-brain power connection. So, he designed a study.

He and his team studied 259 third and fourth graders (8 – 11 years old). The students were measured for physical fitness levels (BMI, flexibility, cardio fitness, etc.). The fitness levels were then checked against their math and reading scores on the statewide Standardized Test.

Sure enough, the fittest kids did the best on these tests. The ones with the fittest bodies had the fittest brains, even with factors such as socioeconomic level taken into account.

This is just one of the many studies proving the sound mind in a sound body anecdote. With new equipment and methods scientists are able to look for the processes...the how of exercise's effect on cognition. There is more evidence and understanding of the complexities of the mind-body connection.

It all starts in the muscles. Every time a muscle contracts it releases a protein called IGF-1 into the blood. This protein travels into the brain itself and initiates the release of several chemicals, one of which is brain-derived neurotrophic factor (BDNF). BDNF fuels almost all the activities leading to higher cognition.

Not only that, but regular exercise causes the body to build up levels of BDNF. The brain's nerve cells branch out and start communicating with one another in new and different ways! In other words, the brain is learning new things. High BDNF = learning. Low BDNF = the brain closes off new learning. Cool!

As adults, most people keep a relatively constant level of BDNF. As we age, individual neurons start to die off. Scientists used to think this was a permanent loss but in the last decade this belief has changed to thinking that parts of the brain can be "re-grown". Exercise is a catalyst. The part of the brain that seems to be most affected by exercise induced growth is the hippocampus, a memory and learning region.

In another study, Professor Author Kramer of the University of Illinois, scanned the frontal lobes of exercisers and found that those areas were affected by exercise too. The frontal lobes are the "higher" thought areas that help with multitasking, decision-making and such.

In addition to BDNF production, exercise creates blood flow to the brain. Just like other parts of the body, regularly increased blood flow grows new capillaries. In the brain where, you have new nerve cells, new capillaries grow to supply the blood.

Of course, the above "neurogenesis" happens with regular exercise. If you are already active, you know that after a hard workout, your brain focus is better and you are calmer. This is the endorphin effect or runner's high that people talk about. The effects of exercise on the brain are immediate and, if maintained, long-lasting.

Who says athletes aren't smart? Not scientists!

Working out is good for the brain.

# The Gym Grunting Controversy

A large well known fitness facility company has a "no grunting" policy. Last year, they made news in the U.S. when they called the police to escort a member out of the gym for grunting. What's the deal with that?

Ok, ok. Aside from being drama queens and a bit annoying, what are these grunters really doing wrong? And how does the gym staff decide what is a grunt and what's just normal exhalation of air upon exertion?

Do they hire "Grunt Monitors"?

I can see it now in Grunt Monitor Training: "Ok grunt monitors, a grunt is considered a legitimate grunt when it sounds like "uuuooooohhhgg" but is not a grunt when it sounds like "ugh"." I mean, honestly – doesn't this seem pretty silly?

Of course, there's the deeper more philosophical question: is there a difference between a snort and a grunt?

What if you drop a weight on your toe and scream "ouch". Do you get expelled for that?

And what are the exact procedures for expulsion from the gym for grunting? Is a member issued a grunt warning first? Maybe two grunt warnings? Three grunts - you are out?

Imagine what happens at the employees' shift change: "Hi Jack, you see that guy over there in the red shirt? Watch him carefully. He's had two grunt warnings already and I believe I heard the beginnings of a grunt earlier. His days are numbered…"

"Ok Susie, you can count on me…I never miss a grunter".

What about the poor grunters? Don't you think they feel discriminated against? Is this the beginning of gym apartheid?

Will people have to be grunt-tested before they can join the gym? If they grunt, will they be sent to the grunter's gym?

New membership drives and advertisements will go something like this: "Are you a grunter?  No problem!  Come on down"  Maybe more avant-garde gyms could have tiered membership fees – as in "Yes indeed sir, we do have a Gold Membership just for grunters.  Of course, it will cost you more."

Most women when they workout make more of a moaning sound than a grunt.  Do gyms need special rules for moaners?

Or is it like ladies night at a bar?  Ladies attract men, so they are allowed to moan.

Here's an idea: they could implement special hours for lady moaners.  That would be good for business, don't you think?  Fit women sweating and making moaning sounds.  Most guys I know would be there for sure – and not to workout either!

On a more serious note, what is the grunting and moaning all about?  Does it really serve any purpose?  Well, there's not much evidence that it serves a physiological purpose.  Psychological?  My guess is that's the reason people do it.

To lift heavy things properly, it's important to breathe deeply.  Holding one's breath when lifting can drive blood pressure up.

There used to be a belief among trainers to teach people to exhale at exertion, but that idea is continuously challenged by new research.  It's more common now for trainers to explain to folks the importance of breathing well and continuously while working out.

Whether one inhales or exhales on the lift doesn't really matter.  Whatever is comfortable is best…so long as breathing occurs.

So here's to all the grunters and moaners out there….happy lifting!

# Let's Compromise...
## Aerobic vs. Anaerobic Training

As a trainer, I often get this question: don't I need to do long duration aerobic training to burn fat? The answer is (drum roll please) both aerobic (low intensity) training and anaerobic (high intensity) training will do the trick. In fact, if you really want to burn fat, include BOTH in your routine.

Let's look at why:

The word aerobic means in the presence of oxygen. Activities performed at low to moderate intensity for around 90 seconds allow oxygen to be used to generate energy for the muscles. An example of this would be brisk walking, slow running or, for us weight lifting aficionados, very low weight high repetition exercises.

Anaerobic activity is any activity where the body does not use oxygen to generate energy. The body uses different metabolic pathways (which I won't bore you with the specifics here) to react to this activity. Anaerobic activities tend to be short duration, burst of activity things where the body just doesn't have time to circulate oxygen to the muscles (less than 90 seconds). Sprints and very heavy low repetition weight lifting are examples of anaerobic exercises.

The benefits of aerobic activity:

1.  Increased cardiovascular endurance
2.  Decreased body fat

The liabilities are:

1.  Decreased muscle mass
2.  Decreased speed
3.  Decreased power

Here's the rub - when the body uses fat for energy it also breaks down muscle. Since muscle cells burn energy and fat cells store it, you need muscle to use energy that would otherwise be stored as fat!

Now, anaerobic training, the kind where you push yourself hard for short periods of time, uses a different metabolic system to supply the muscles with energy, which trains the body to respond in a different way to exercise.

The benefits of Anaerobic Training are:

1. Increased Cardiovascular Capacity
2. Increased Cardiovascular Recovery Ability
3. Strength Gains
4. Power Gains
5. Improved Speed
6. Decreased Body Fat

The liabilities:

1. Increased Risk of Injury in Untrained People
2. Requires a Good Aerobic Foundation

When we look at all of the elements of fitness, which include:

- Endurance

- Strength

- Flexibility

- Power

- Speed

- Agility

- Balance

It's easy to see why a combination of aerobic and anaerobic training will do the most for your fitness level. And, since both aerobic and anaerobic training burn fat (anaerobic training actually yields the most post workout fat burning), the combining the two in your routine will burn fat and maintain muscle. Not only will you burn fat faster, you will keep the fat off and won't be bored in the process!

# Fitness: The Great Equalizer

One of the most rewarding things about being a fitness trainer is empowering someone to accomplish their goals and watching them do it. Everyone has a different reason for embracing a fitness lifestyle, but the outcomes are pretty much always the same. The person feels better and has more confidence because the body they live in is vibrant, healthy and able. One thing's for sure, mentoring someone to transform is great fun.

My husband Dave and I live in an interesting community. It is full of "expats" (people who do not live in their home culture). As such, my fitness clients are from everywhere. This makes for interesting communication challenges and requires some different mentoring and leadership skills. One group that I have is a group of young Japanese women who don't speak much English and I, unfortunately, have very little Japanese. We use lots of body language! Oops, I digress.

Getting to the idea that fitness is a "great equalizer". What does this mean? It means that doing it means getting better at it. This applies to everyone – no matter what level they start from. As an example, I currently have 2 clients that joined me about the same time. Both are women. One is 55 and has always been sedentary except for light housework and walking. The other is a thirty year old dancer who became overweight over a period of about 10 years. The older lady is motivated because she is having health problems from her lack of activity and extra body fat. The younger lady is motivated to become leaner and stay active.

When I met the older client, I thought she was much older than her years by the way she moved and the way she talked about what she could and couldn't do. When she started exercising, she moved slowly. Her joints were stiff and her brain to body communication was slow. She started at level one. Within weeks, however, she was moving well and fluently. She has since reported that her blood pressure is lower and she says she feels so much better. This week in step aerobics class she was keeping up with the much younger participants!

The younger client is really seeing body changes and feeling different. She is leaner and has a radiance to her skin that is remarkable. She plans to run a 10K race in 2 months. She is looking good and feeling good!

The great equalizer: Both started about 2 months ago. Both are consistently exercising and making healthier food choices. Both are beginning to see and feel results after 2 months – within the scope and realistic expectations that they had when they began.

The greatest thing to witness through this transformation is what I like to call "the side effects". When I talk to both of these ladies about what they are doing, I feel their happiness and their sense of empowerment about taking charge of their own health. It is hard work, but the rewards are tangible and visible. The changes are emotional as well as physical!

Last night Dave and I were talking about his fitness "transformation". You see, he decided 7 years ago (age 41) that, although he was exercising and eating well, he wasn't as fit as he would like to be. So he embarked on a journey of transformation. He was so excited about his change that he wrote a book about it! He and I started dating after he had "transformed". I said to him that I am not sure I would have dated him if he didn't keep himself fit.

Ok, ok... even I'll admit that this sounds superficial, but for me it's not. Why? Although I DO appreciate a man (or woman) with a fit body - it's much more than that. A person who keeps him or herself fit has an aura about them - a sense of empowerment about their own health and body. And let's face it, empowered people are attractive people!

So, congratulations to all of you out there who have recently made the decision to embrace a fitness lifestyle. Enjoy the journey!

# Get Fit, Not Hurt

How many of you have had this experience? There's been no time to get to the gym in the last month or so. So finally when there is time, you (consciously or subconsciously) "make up" for lost time. The next day…OUCH, you feel like you've been hit by a truck!

This is a common scenario for most of us. New exercisers often "overdo" at first because they are unaware of the impact of sudden and intense activity on the body and its need for adjustment.

Regular and experienced exercisers often forget that fitness slowly declines when stopped for more than a couple of weeks. The body needs to readjust to the demands placed on it. For me, it's just plain old ego…I don't want to admit to myself that I have lost any of my fitness!

"Overdoing" is just one of the many ways that we can hurt ourselves when we are using our bodies vigorously. Aside from the obvious twisted ankle (acute injury), there are many injuries that happen insidiously (tendonitis, arthritis etc.). Now before I scare you away from exercise, its worth mentioning that most of these injuries happen just as often in sedentary people because of lack of exercise.

So, the real point of this chapter is to give you some guidelines to help you avoid exercise/sports injuries whether you are a newbie or an experienced exerciser/sports participant:

- Wear proper shoes for the particular sport or activity.

- Always were protective gear for the sports you are involved in. Helmets are not just for kids!

- Comfortable clothes that you can move in are always good, but special outfits for the sport are not usually required unless you like them or if they are for a team.

- Start out slowly if you are new to the sport or exercise OR you haven't done it in more than 2 weeks.

- Warm up BEFORE stretching. This is important. Muscles are tight when cold and stretching them can injure them. What is a good warm up? A slower version of the activity you are going to do is good. For example, walk for 5 minutes before you begin running. If you are going to throw a ball, gentle arm circles and other movements for several minutes will warm up the shoulder and elbow joints.

- Stretch often. Stretching can be performed after warm-up, but I find it to be the most efficient when I am finished with the activity or when there's a break in the activity. The muscles are warm and most receptive. Always be careful not to overstretch.

- Take lessons or training if you are new to the activity. This ensures that you are moving in such a way to not only perform well (win!) but also not injure yourself. I have personal experience with this: I decided to run a marathon. I trained myself but just couldn't accomplish the distances I needed to get there. Then, I had coaching for my running style which I was told was a speed style, not distance style. I thought running was something we all do naturally and all that's needed to run was to run! Since that coaching, I have completed many marathons.

- Add new activities or exercises carefully. The body needs time to adapt.

- Drink LOTS of fluid (water is usually best) before, during and after your activity, especially in hot weather. A good guide for this is 500ml of liquid every 15 minutes during the activity. The body needs water both before and after exercise and during it as well. You will find your performance to be much better!

- Apply the 10% rule. This is a great rule of thumb. Increase your time OR intensity level by a maximum of 10% per week. If you are running, increase either distance by 10% per week or speed by 10% per week – but not both in the same week. If you are weight lifting, increase the number of times you lift the weight (repetitions) by 10% maximum or the amount of weight by 10% maximum per week.

- If you are already working with injuries, talk to your physical therapist or personal trainer about what to do that works and doesn't work with your body and situation.

Listen to your body! If you are tired, rest! If you have pain beyond muscle soreness or swelling, see a doctor.

# Exercise for Physical, Emotional and Intellectual Fitness

In July, my daughter and I went snow skiing (yes, I did say July - southern hemisphere winter). During the week we skied, both of us took lots of lessons. My daughter because she is new to skiing and me because the last time I skied was 18 years ago! Those of you who ski know that the way one skis is different than it used to be because the design of the skis has changed. Easier in many ways once you embrace the differences!

Anyway, the instructor that I had said something that really stuck with me... and hence this chapter. He said "it takes 1000 repetitions of a movement to make it become automatic". If you are involved in a sport, performing art or other physically based pursuit, this will make a lot of sense to you. As a dancer and fitness instructor, I see this in action a lot. Rehearsing for a show, ideally one rehearses to the point where the body takes over on stage. If the movements are automatic, you can emotionally freeze up (stage fright), engage the audience or even think about other things and your body will do it anyway. When this happens, for me this feels as if my head has detached from my body and is having a great time!

So what is the point being made here? The brain makes new neural pathways for each new movement that we do. It grows much in the same way as when you play a mathematics game or do any new intellectual activity. Also, when you use these new physical movement skills in different ways, the brain has to develop ways to access these movements from memory and sequence them.

Given this, it stands to reason that doing not only exercises you enjoy but also a variety of exercises leads to better health and a more flexible brain at all life stages. After all, we insist our kids expose themselves to sports, games, math, music, languages, drama (ok, too long but you get the idea) to help them grow and develop!

So, let's say that you have a routine that has gotten you fit and you like it because it works within your life goals and restrictions. (Life can get in the way of one's fitness activities!) For example, on Mondays, Wednesdays and Fridays you like to go for a run early in the morning. Tuesdays and Thursdays you work out with weights at home. It makes you feel good, you like it and you don't want to change. Don't! But how about "tweaking" your runs to include other things? Or incorporate different types of running, such as sprinting into your routine? In the case of your weight workout, how about varying the speed of each lift? Small changes seem simple enough, but my guess is your brain will resist at first - it will "feel" weird.

Now, let's look at the link between brain fitness and emotional well-being. I think you will agree that brain health and emotional health are connected. I mean, how clearly do you think under extreme stress? Some years ago, I was seeing a psychotherapist because I felt I needed help coping with the stress of some life changes I was making. One of the things I learned is that an emotionally healthy person is flexible and less fearful of change. The more stressed or fearful we are the more we tend to try to control the situations we put ourselves into. Add this idea to the knowledge that we have of exercise improving mood and helping with depression (runner's high or whatever you want to name it) and what conclusions can we make?

- Moving your body builds new neural pathways.

- Physical movements build different neural pathways as do intellectual activities.

- Stress causes physical as well as emotional responses in the body and the brain.

- Exercising increases the feel good hormones in the body.

- Exercise helps with physical manifestations of emotions like sleep problems, lack of appetite and nervousness.

- A stressed or fearful person doesn't handle change well.

- The brain, like the body can become less flexible with age unless it is used (the old anecdote that "you can't teach an old dog new tricks").

- Physical activity improves mental acuity, emotional well being and brain flexibility.

My personal conclusion....Adding or changing fitness activities or taking up new sports appears to be yet another way to keep our brains (and bodies) fitter, younger and help us be more confident when presented with stressors associated with life's challenges.

# Experience is a Great Motivator

Do you know the saying, "We are all a product of our experiences"?

If you have gone through a major life change or trauma which created the physical symptoms of anxiety or grief, you understand how physically uncomfortable this can be with stomach aches, elevated heart rates and such. Not only do these symptoms happen at the time; but often months or years later, a memory of the event can trigger these symptoms again. These are strong emotions associated with big events.

Most of us like to avoid uncomfortable feelings whenever possible, right?

With life altering events, it's easy to recognize memories and events that "trigger" bad feelings. The emotions are strong and hence the physical response is strong as well. But what about lesser events?

AND…What does this have to do with fitness? Ok, Ok…I'm getting there!

Let's say you are a 35 year old man who was an athlete in High School. You developed a nice athletic body that has served you well. But lately, you are feeling like you look a bit "soft" and feel sluggish. So you decide that you should work on your body some.

So, off to the gym. After all, you used to be very fit, so it should be easy to get it back. You enter the gym. It's big, busy and intimidating. But, the people working out don't look like professional body builders, just normal people. You begin to feel comfortable.

Since it's your first time at the gym, you are assigned a Fitness Trainer to help you get started. You don't really need help, you tell yourself…after all you are in pretty good shape for 35. The trainer helps you to a treadmill and asks you to walk for 5 minutes to warm up. Instead of walking, you jog. It hasn't been that long since high school, has it?

After that, the trainer takes you through a series of machines and free weights and explains how to use them and what weight levels to start with. The trainer then hands you your card record, wishes you luck and encourages you to ask for help anytime. Off you go...

Now the moment of truth: you are worn out from the treadmill, and barely strong enough to do the weight levels and exercises on your card! After a few minutes, you feel so tired, discouraged and even embarrassed because all the people around you suddenly seem to be SO much stronger and more accomplished than you.

The next day, you are too sore to move! An emotionally negative experience for sure.

There are 2 ways to go here: you can tell yourself that it's just not for you. This way, you don't have to go back and face those negative feelings again. OR you can use those emotions to galvanize you to action!

Fitness is what I like to call a "great equalizer". In other words, if you do it, you get stronger and better. If you don't do it, you will not get stronger and better.

Like painting a house, each trip to the gym is another coat of paint. It gets easier both physically and emotionally with each workout. Very quickly, it feels good to be there. Then it feels good to see changes and get stronger. Then, you start seeking the next challenge with excitement.

Not to mention that after a while, you start to make friends at the gym and feel a part of something.

I have used a gym workout as an example, but the same holds true for the sports you choose to be involved in. You do it, you get the physical benefits. Getting the physical benefits leads to positive emotions. The positive emotions motivate you to repeat the experience rather than avoid it. Repeating the experience causes you to get fitter which brings more positive emotions...and so on.

So, if you are having trouble starting or staying with a fitness activity, take a visit inside yourself to see if past experiences and emotions are holding you back. You might be surprised what you learn.

# NUTRITION

# What in the World is a Crossover Food?

Looking for healthy, inexpensive and versatile ways to add more protein into your diet?

Why not consider dried beans?

Dried beans, also known as legumes and pulses, are not only a great source of protein, but are low in fat, packed with vitamins, minerals and both soluble and insoluble fiber.

Ask any vegetarian how they get enough protein in their diet and they probably will say "I eat a lot of beans".

I decided to become a vegetarian as a small child and my parents (who were not vegetarians by the way) worried that I would be lacking in the protein necessary for growth. So, after consulting with my pediatrician and many books on raising vegetarian children, they added beans and lentils to the family table. Not only did I grow, but I am the tallest woman in my family, an enormous 5 feet 5 inches tall. Yea, well, my family is not famous for its tall women.

## Protein, Fiber, Vitamins and Minerals

Ok, ok, back to the beans. Beans are an excellent, non-fat source of protein. Just one cup of beans has about 16 grams, about the same as 3 ounces (audio cassette size) piece of chicken, fish or beef.

Because they are a plant, they contain fiber, vitamins and minerals like vegetables. Nutritionists refer to them as "crossover foods" which means they can be used in a meal as a protein or vegetable item. Take a look at the cuisines of different countries and cultures. You will notice that most cultures include beans, prepared in many different ways. Such a versatile food!

Another unique quality of beans is the fiber. Beans contain both soluble and insoluble fiber. Huh? What does this mean?

Insoluble fiber is the technical term for what my Mom always referred to as "roughage". You know.. the stuff that makes food move through your body more easily. Insoluble fiber has received a lot of publicity in recent years because of the link to a high fiber diet and lowered risk of several types of cancer.

Soluble fiber forms a "gooey" substance in the digestive process that helps with processing of fats, cholesterol and slows the release of carbohydrates into the bloodstream. The American Diabetic Association loves beans!

Beans are rich in antioxidants, folic acid, vitamin B-6 and magnesium. Folic Acid and B-6 are known for their ability to lower homocysteine levels in the blood.

Elevated blood levels of homocysteine in the blood are associated with risk for heart attack, stroke and peripheral vascular disease. 20-40 percent of patients with heart disease have elevated homocysteine levels.

So, what's the downside of this wonderful food? If you are not used to a high fiber diet….flatulence. As with the introduction of any high fiber food, go easy with the amounts the first few days until your body adjusts. Then any uncomfortable feeling will probably pass.

## How to Cook

You can use canned beans which are nutritionally similar to dried ones. It's a good idea to rinse the beans before eating them to remove the salt and preservatives used in canning.

I tend to try and avoid processed foods where possible so I buy dried beans and cook them following the instructions on the package. Generally, beans are not complicated to cook, but require time. Most beans, except lentils, require an overnight soak in water to soften them up. Then they can be simmered until soft on the stove or in a slow cooker. Generally, the bigger the bean, the longer they take to cook. One thing to note: after soaking, rinse the beans and cook them in new water. This will help prevent flatulence!

Beans can be frozen after cooking and used in sauces, soups, salads or anywhere your imagination takes you. Where I live, red bean ice cream is popular. Delicious!

# Natural is not the Same as Organic

Organic foods have become very popular in recent times. I haven't been in a MacDonald's lately, but I bet there's even an organic selection on their menu! Personally, I get a warm and fuzzy feeling knowing that the entree I order is organic or do I? Wait a minute! What does "organic" really mean and why does organic food cost so much more?

In an endeavor to answer this question, I looked up the United States Department of Agriculture (USDA) guidelines on raising food that receives the "USDA certified organic" seal of approval.

The rules go something like this:

- The land has to be free for 3 years before growing from certain prohibited substances which include sewage sludge (oh man! Does this mean non-organic farmers use sewage sludge?).

- The farmers can't use genetic engineering or ionizing radiation.

- The organic foods and the non-organic foods cannot be processed together or come in contact with chemicals.

- Livestock must be fed 100% organic feed.

- Livestock cannot be given hormones or antibiotics.

- Livestock must have outdoor access.

This is informative, but doesn't give the whole picture as to what organic is. The term "organic" refers to the way that farmers grow, handle and process our food. Organic is a philosophy of farming where "conventional methods" of fertilization, weed control and livestock disease prevention are used. Farmers use natural fertilizers like manure, try where possible to use beneficial insects and birds instead of pesticides, rotate crops, weed by hand and feed livestock organic feed.

Natural does not necessarily mean organic. However, there are some other terms, types of growing and husbandry methods that might be important to you such as "free-range" or "hormone free".

Whether you buy organic or not, the USDA also recommends eating many different kinds of fruit, vegetables, meat and dairy. This is not only to ensure that you get the most nutrients possible from your food, but also to keep from saturating your system with the same chemicals (pesticides, herbicides, hormones, antibiotics and fertilizers).

Even if you don't choose organic, it's always a good  idea to wash and scrub your vegetables/fruit with a brush. This will remove more chemical residues than washing alone. Better yet, peel them when you can!

Take care of your body!

# Isn't Vegan a Planet in the Next Solar System?

Forty years ago, when I was a kid (and a vegetarian newbie), vegetarianism was not common. The statement "I am a vegetarian" was met with a simple "Oh". Then came the 1980s when it became fashionable to be vegetarian for health reasons. With this fashion came confusion...

If you are a long term vegetarian like me, you will no doubt have been asked "Do you eat chicken and fish?" Answer: polite yet emphatic "No, I am a vegetarian". This question is usually followed by "How do you get enough protein?" Answer: polite yet emphatic "Easy!"

For those that are confused, here's a brief description of the types of vegetarianism. Basically, there are those who either eat dairy (lacto vegetarian), eggs (ovo vegetarian) or both (ovo-lacto vegetarian). Vegans are vegetarians that consume no animal products at all. Among us vegetarians, if we say we are vegetarian it is taken to mean we eat dairy and or eggs. Vegans usually use the word vegan, which sounds to me like terminology invented by the producers of the original Star Trek episodes.

This chapter is about vegetarian and vegan eating, either as a lifestyle or the occasional meal. This chapter is about eating for muscle development. Is it possible to do both? Yes it is... with simple foods and a bit of knowledge about the composition of proteins.

Amino acids are the building blocks of protein. To build or maintain muscle (and most other body functions), the human body requires some amino acids that it must take from food. These are called the Essential Amino Acids. There are other amino acids that the body manufactures on its own – called Non-essential Amino Acids. However, it requires the essential ones to manufacture the non-essential ones.

A protein is referred to as "complete" or "useable" when it contains all of the essential amino acids. Animal protein is complete. Vegetables, fruits, beans, nuts and seeds all contain protein, but they usually are not complete and therefore need to be "complemented" with foods that have the missing amino acids. The exception to this is soybeans. The protein in soybeans is complete and needs no complement.

In a nutshell: for vegetarians, getting enough protein is as simple as eating eggs, dairy products and soybeans products (except soy sauce) - all of which are good sources of high quality "useable" protein. For vegans, dried beans and soy are the main source of protein. Dried beans need to be complemented with nuts, grains, corn, eggs, dairy or soy (except eggs and dairy for vegans). For Non-vegetarians, a small amount of meat, fish or chicken in a meal will also complete the protein in beans or nuts for an extra protein punch that's also packed with phytochemicals and anti-oxidants!

Live long and prosper.

# Not All Carbohydrates
# are Created Equal

"You might as well eat the box. It has more nutrition than the cereal inside". These are the words of my mother every morning when I was a kid.

Of course, that was the 1960s which was the real beginning of the popularity of pre-prepared convenience foods. Nutrition science was more geared toward preventing beri beri than promoting health and longevity.

Nutrition science has come a long way since then and provides you new tools such as the Glycemic Index (GI) and the Glycemic Load (GL).

## What is the Glycemic Index (GI)?

The Glycemic Index is a ranking of foods based on how they affect blood glucose (sugar) levels. Since protein and fat don't really impact blood glucose, it's really an index of the rate that carbohydrates are broken down in the gut and enter the bloodstream. The higher the GI number, the faster it goes into the blood.

Eating high GI foods triggers an insulin mechanism which causes the body to store fat. For most of us, eating a lot of high GI foods causes an increase in fat storage.

Most beans, whole grains and non-starchy vegetables have a low glycemic index; while sugars, foods made from refined flour (eg., white bread), most fruits and some root vegetables have a high GI.

The more processed, cooked or chewed a food is, the higher the GI because the gut doesn't have much to break down. Soluble fiber, like in beans slows down the release of carbohydrates in the blood. The degree of ripeness of a fruit: more ripe = higher GI. Acidic foods, like lemon juice and vinegar slow release of sugar. Salty foods increase the rate of release. Protein in a meal will lower the overall GI of the whole meal.

## What is the Glycemic Load (GL)?

Now, if you take a look on the web at one of the many glycemic index listings available, you will notice that carrots have a very high GI - almost as much as sugar! That does seem a bit odd. Enter the concept of glycemic load index (GL).

The GL takes into account not only the type of sugar (how quickly it spikes blood sugar) but also the amount of other stuff in the food that doesn't affect blood sugar - like water and fiber. There is a mathematical calculation which I won't bore you with.

For example, a half-cup serving of carrots has a GI of 131 (very high) but since it is mostly fiber and water has only 6.2 grams of carbs. The glycemic load of that portion size is 6 (low GL). By contrast, a plain five-ounce bagel has a GI of 72 (high) and has 65 grams of carbohydrate. Its glycemic load is very high at 47.

## How Is This Useful?

The GL index is a recent development and is still mostly used by diabetics to balance the blood sugar release of whole meals. The GI, which was developed in the early 1980s, helps diabetics manage nutrition, but endurance athletes also use it for "Carbo Loading". It is common for athletes to use low and medium GI foods before an event and high GI foods during and after the event to fuel the muscles quickly for recovery.

The Bottom Line?

Eating low on the GI is an easy way for all of us who want to keep our body efficiently using fat rather than storing it and to keep our energy levels consistent throughout the day.

Happy and healthy eating!

# The Bigger, the Better?

In the last 10 years or so, we have seen the advent of "supersized" foods. And quite honestly some of the supersized products are so big they are ridiculous… and it looks like they are still getting bigger. But are these extra big products affecting the size of our bodies or is it all just hype?

I just returned from a holiday where I visited 2 countries. For the purposes of this chapter, I will call the countries, Country 1 and Country 2. Both Country 1 and 2 are in the same region of the world with basically the same good quality food and culturally healthy diets. Lots of fruit, veggies, lean meats simply prepared and dairy. Yet, my traveling companion and I both noticed a sizeable difference in the "fatness" of the populations of the 2 countries. What gives?

As a tourist, I ate in restaurants and therefore wasn't exposed to the normal day to day eating habits and cultural mores surrounding food and mealtimes in these countries. But one thing really stood out in the restaurants as being a possible culprit…. portion sizes.

Country 1: ENORMOUS plates of food served in the restaurants

Country 2: Small/normal sized plates of food served in the restaurants.

Up to now, I haven't paid much attention to portion sizing as a possible reason that people become overweight, but this observation peaked my interest.

So, upon returning home to my computer I did some surfing on the subject of portion sizing and weight management. Do you know that they have a name for the psychological impact of portion sizing on eating habits? It's called "unit bias".

Apparently, there's been lots of studies to determine whether people are affected by the size of the food itself as well as the utensils and container sizes the food is in. One of my personal favorites is the M&M study. The researchers put a large jar of M&Ms out in a public area. They changed the scoopers to a different size each day. Low and behold, on the days where the smaller scoopers were used, people took fewer M&Ms. The conclusion here is that the people judged a "serving" to be whatever the size of the scooper was.

Getting back to my trip. It's interesting to observe that people of different cultures do have different ideas of what is "enough" food. For example, my traveling companion on this trip is originally from Country 1 (the one with big portions). While traveling in Country 2 after a week in Country 1, he kept commenting on how he would have to order double to get enough to eat. I noticed that in Country 1, I was so overwhelmed by the large plates of food that I started ordering only 1 item and I still ate until my stomach hurt. In Country 2, like my traveling companion, I felt the need to order more than 1 item each meal (I also put on a kilo of fat in 2 weeks!)

So, for me this idea has become much more evident. Portion sizes are a matter of perception...a perception that can be detrimental to our health and body shape. So if you are always struggling with extra fat, take a look at the size of your plates!

# The United Colors of....Fruits and Vegetables!

Years ago, a good friend of mine, Dan, told me something that I have used over and over again with clients when explaining simple ways to eat healthily. Dan is someone who reads a fair bit and thinks about the logic of things. Hence, he takes care of himself by following solid nutrition principles and exercising regularly. Pretty wise guy all around.

So, back to Dan's comment: He said something like (it was a long time ago so I can't quote him exactly), "I read a nutrition recommendation that really made sense to me. It said to try and eat as many different colors everyday as you can". At the time, it struck me as very powerful and simple. Do you know why? Antioxidants!

"Antioxidants" is quite the buzz word in the world of nutrition these days. This is because cellular oxidation is a mechanism of aging and related diseases in which nutrition and lifestyle choices play a part.

Oxygen radicals, or free radicals, are a normal part of our body's functioning. Even though we all have them in our body at any given time, they cause cellular damage. This is called oxidation. In our bodies, this process is similar to the process that happens to unpainted metal after a time…it rusts and deteriorates. To stop rust on metal, you add oil or paint. But what's the best way to slow it in our bodies?

If our body has a way to absorb the oxygen radicals, they don't do damage.

What's the best way to absorb free radicals? Eat LOTS of richly colored vegetables and fruits. Simple.

Of course, some vegetables and fruits are better at absorbing free radicals. I was curious about this idea, so I checked out the web for more information. What

I found confirmed my thinking that, as a rule the richer and deeper the color, the more powerful the antioxidant actions in the body.

The United States Department of Agriculture developed a test, called the Oxygen Radical Absorbance Capacity or ORAC (could they make the name any longer??), which assigns a score to each vegetable depending on it's antioxidant capacity.   And, YEP, sure enough, with a few exceptions like garlic and cauliflower, the deeper colored veggies and fruits had higher scores.

If you are interested to learn about specific veggies and fruits that you like, search for "ORAC scores of fruits and vegetables" in your web search engine. There's tons of information out there. I have listed a couple of sites below that are good as well.

OR just follow Dan's philosophy and eat as many colors as you can everyday. Your body will love you for it. THANKS Dan!

# The Vitamin D Debates Continue

I was doing some research on a topic that my brother-in-law, an MD who works in university research, mentioned to me over the holidays. Every time I see this guy, he always gives me ideas! I came across a startling introduction to an article written by John Cannell which I thought I would steal:

What rat poison is safer than water?

The answer is ... Vitamin D.

Turns out, there's a lot of new research on this vitamin and, as my brother in law said, the research is indicating that many of us need much more of this vitamin than we are getting. Apparently, vitamin D plays a role in the prevention of much more than just bone loss. Receptors for vitamin D are found in most of the cells of the body. It has been shown to contribute to a healthy immune system, muscle strength and hormone production.

The major function of vitamin D is to maintain normal blood levels of calcium and phosphorus. Vitamin D aids in the absorption of calcium, helping to form and maintain strong bones. Recent research also suggests it may provide protection from osteoporosis, hypertension, heart disease, certain cancers and several autoimmune diseases including diabetes.

But here's speculation that I found really interesting: vitamin D may help in weight control. You might have heard of the study that cites that folks with more calcium in their diets tended to have lower body mass indices (BMI). Well, given that vitamin D is responsible for controlling calcium levels in the blood, it follows that this vitamin plays a role in the high calcium, low BMI phenomenon.

Researchers have also found that obese people have an impaired ability to synthesize vitamin D from sunlight. And, they are looking into the connection between excess calcium deposits in the arteries (cardiovascular disease) and low blood levels of vitamin D. Hmmm..

Vitamin D also plays a role in blood sugar regulation. Swings in blood sugar signal our body's fat storage mechanism and signals our brain to eat or not.

Don't we get vitamin D from sunlight?

Vitamin D is often called the sunshine vitamin because the body synthesizes it from sunlight - specifically, from UV-B rays. Yep, these are the ones we know as the burning rays. In places further from the equator, these rays are most available between 10 am and 2 pm. Most of us avoid spending much time in the sun at these times because we get sunburned which increases our risk of skin cancer and premature skin aging. UV-B rays are blocked well by sunscreens and by glass (glass doesn't block UV-As). Depending on the pigment in your skin, it takes different bodies different amounts of time in the midday sun to get adequate levels of vitamin D. The darker your skin, the more time you need in the sun to get enough of the vitamin.

So, now on to dietary vitamin D: Cod Liver Oil has a lot of vitamin D, followed by some oily fishes, lard (pork fat), butter, dairy fat and egg yolks. Beyond that, it's pretty difficult to get enough of this vitamin from dietary sources alone. So, if you work inside and wear sunscreen, or live at latitudes far from the equator, supplementation may a good thing.

But even supplementation recommendations are now under fire by the researchers. The most common recommendations that I have seen is 400 IU per day for kids, 200 IU per day for adults under 50 years old and 400 IU per day for those over 50. Some researchers are advocating MUCH higher doses – in the 1000 IU to 2000 IU per day range! There is even a lot of debate about toxicity levels of this vitamin among them. Some say more that 2000 IU per day can be toxic, some say 20,000 IU per day is not!

I took a look at my super-duper Women's Multivitamin that I buy at the health food store. It yields 400 IU per day. I am 47 years old, live on the equator where there's lots of UV-B rays much of the day, but work mostly inside and do wear sunscreen every day. So, I have decided to be on the safe side to increase my daily dose of vitamin D supplements to 600-800 IU. This is below what researchers are saying but above recommendations for my age. Remember that when looking at this vitamin, it's important to keep in mind the amount of midday sun exposure you normally get on average, how far you live from the equator, how dark your skin is and how much vitamin D your multivitamin supplies.

Of course, I will keep checking in with my brother in law and published research to keep track of any updates....and will keep you posted.

# The Longevity Diet?

Have you heard of the Longevity Diet or Calorie Restriction Diet? It's been in and out of nutrition news for many years; the theory and related research starting in the 1930s. The concept is that by eating less total calories and ensuring that the calories we do eat are highly nutritious, we can extend our life span. So what's the science behind this? No one knows exactly, but the research is growing, and so are the numbers of people trying it out.

In the 1930s, researchers studying growth patterns and food deprivation in mice noticed that adult mice that were underfed lived much longer than their well fed counterparts. Since then, there have been studies done on different animals, including primates, with basically the same results: those animals that were fed much fewer "high quality" calories lived longer and had better overall health.

Do you remember Biosphere 2? It was the project where they built a sealed, self-contained facility in Arizona and people lived there for 2 years. Well, the food production part of the experiment didn't go so well yet the participants stayed anyway. It was observed that although they became very thin, their health profiles (particularly the biomarkers of aging: cholesterol, blood sugar and c-reactive protein/inflammation) improved considerably.

This led to the formation of the Calorie Restriction Society by one of the Biosphere 2 members, Dr. Roy Walford. The society aims to raise money for research as well as to educate people on the benefits and risks of Calorie Restriction as a lifestyle. They have renamed the concept: Calorie Restriction with Optimal Nutrition. This is an important distinction, because if one restricts their calories from between 10 to 30%, it is imperative that what is eaten is high quality in terms of nutrition. No junk food allowed!

What researchers have found are the benefits of Calorie Restriction with Optimal Nutrition? Well, in humans it's not an easy research study to design because we live so long and there aren't many people willing to go to such extremes. But there have been some interesting findings.

This year, a research group studied 25 members of the Calorie Restriction Society (aged 41-65) who had been following the lifestyle eating 1400 to 2000 calories per day for an average of 6 years, along with another 25 people who had been eating "normal" American diet of 2,000 to 3,000 calories per day. They measured the diastolic function of all of them. This is a biomarker of age in hearts. The calorie restrictors' diastolic readings were of people 15 years younger.

One research group has been able to prove that calorie restriction in mice slows down death rates, particularly of cancer and kidney failure. Well fed, sedentary lab rats commonly die of these afflictions. They demonstrated that calorie restriction slows down the growth speed of breast, skin and white blood cells... which means a slower tumor growth rate.

One researcher is studying the implications of the fact that calorie restriction lowers the levels of insulin and insulin growth factor –another cancer trigger. This also can't be bad in the fight for diabetes prevention and control!

And yet another research group is studying the idea that slowing down the amount of energy given to the mitochondria of our cells gives us fewer free radicals (cellular respiration generates free radicals). Hmm... many of us are taking anti-oxidant vitamins to combat free radical damage – maybe we just need to eat less.

Although the concept really hasn't been studied enough to lend concrete answers, it deserves the attention of those of us who are looking to live longer and more productive lives. Many of the principles put forth by this lifestyle, such as to eat more nutrient dense foods (veggies, fruits, lean dairy, fish, lean meats and whole grains) and eat fewer empty calories (sugar, white flour, white rice and other processed foods), couldn't be bad for anyone!

It's pretty obvious that being overweight is a risk factor for a shortened lifespan, so why wouldn't being mildly underweight lengthen lifespan? It's an idea well worth consideration.

# The Many Disguises of Mono Sodium Glutamate

The other day, I got an email from an American guy who lives in Malaysia. He was saying that cooking with mono sodium glutamate (MSG) is a real health problem to Malaysians and that he "doesn't allow it in his house".

MSG, so what's the big deal? It's the stuff used in large quantities in Chinese/Southeast Asian food, right? Wrong. It's everywhere in almost all processed foods! You see, it was derived from seaweed in Japan in the 1930s and very quickly became popular in United States as a food additive. As long ago as the 1970s, manufacturers promised to take it out of baby food because of suspected problems – no kidding.

Consumers long ago became savvy to MSG listed as an ingredient on food labels and stopped buying things with MSG. So guess what? Manufacturers just renamed the stuff. Here are some of the ingredient names in food that are "cover names" for MSG:

Broth
Casein or Caseinate
Glutamate
Hydrolyzed Yeast
Autolyzed Yeast
Yeast Extract
Hydrolyzed Protein
Natural Flavors

MSG is one of the most popular food additives in food in the US. Fast food chains and restaurants use a lot of it. McDonald's uses it to flavor French fries, the Grilled Chicken Fillet and the Sausage Patties. Pizza Hut uses it to flavor their Chicken Wings. In the supermarket, you can bet that if it's a sauce, salad dressing, snack foods, potato, tortilla chips, soups, crackers, cookies it's probably got MSG in it. It's everywhere – even baby formula. If it's a processed or "convenience" food, it's likely to have MSG. Why?

Because people buy stuff that tastes good.

The science: Have you heard of glutamic acid or glutamate? It's a naturally occurring amino acid in foods. MSG is the sodium salt extracted from glutamic acid. Originally, MSG was derived from protein rich foods, like seaweed; but now it's made from starch, corn sugar, molasses or sugar beets. Well, glutamate naturally occurring in foods is a bound amino acid and the body is equipped to process it as other protein. But, when processed, it becomes free and the body processes it differently.

Simply put, high levels of unbound glutamate causes free radical damage throughout the body. So, eating a lot of processed protein foods where the glutamic acid has been "unbound" results in free radical damage – which is host to all sorts of diseases, most notably cancer. MSG falls into this category. And since it tastes so good, people want more and more of it. Other processed protein foods which end up with free glutamic acids include: ultra pasteurized milk, (this is an unlikely one) the wax they put on vegetables and fruit, which contains hydrolyzed protein and ultra pasteurized soy milk.

Another side note: MSG is an excitotoxin. When consumed, it excites brain neurons so much that they are damaged or even die! Aspartame, sold in the U.S. as NutraSweet and Europe as Candarel is also classified as an excitotoxin. Yuk.

What to do? Well, I suppose we as consumers have to vote with our purchases. Armed with the knowledge that food manufacturers and restaurants are using MSG and disguising it; we need to read labels, ask questions and stop buying products that will harm us.

Eat well, stay healthy!

# Dietary Fats…The Good, Bad and the Ugly

We have all been hearing a lot lately about our Omega-3 fatty acid to Omega-6 ratios and how the typical western diet has "flipped" the ratio backwards. Basically, we eat too many omega-6, not enough omega-3 and too much saturated and trans fat. Omega-3 fatty acids are sorely lacking in the typical western diet, having been replaced by oils with a high proportion of omega-6 oils such as corn oil.

So what does all this mean?

The fats in foods are a combination of saturated, monounsaturated and polyunsaturated. Omega-3 and 6 fats are polyunsaturated. All oils and fats contain a combination of the above. But, some fats have a higher proportion of saturates (butter) or monounsaturates (olive oil) or polyunsaturates (nut oils, corn oil, etc.).

Trans fats are produced when an oil is "hydrogenated". More simply, the oils are processed to make them more stable and less likely to go rancid quickly. Trans fats are used in most processed foods and are not good for the body. Vegetable shortening is hydrogenated oil – lots of trans fats!

With the exception of trans fats, the body requires all of the above fatty acids in different combinations. Yes – even saturated fats. These fatty acids are used to help the body absorb vitamins such as Vitamin A as well as a host of processes like cellular metabolism and the manufacture of hormone-like substances.

Alpha-linolenic acid is one of two fatty acids traditionally classified as "essential." The other fatty acid traditionally known as "essential" is an omega 6 fat called linoleic acid. "Essential" means that the body is unable to manufacture them on its own and they must come from the diet.

The body converts alpha-linolenic acid into two important omega 3 fats, eicosapentaenoic acid (EPA) and docosahexaenoic acid (DHA). EPA plays a role in the prevention of cardiovascular disease, while DHA is the necessary for proper brain and nerve development.

Omega 3 fats also play a role in the production of hormone-like substances called prostaglandins. Prostaglandins help regulate many functions like blood pressure, blood clotting, nerve transmission, inflammation, allergic responses, kidney function, gastrointestinal function and the production of other hormones.

Depending on the type of fat in the diet, certain types of prostaglandins may be produced in large quantities, while others may not be produced at all. This can lead to an imbalance in the body and ....disease.

From omega-3 fats are manufactured series 3 prostaglandins, which act to reduce platelet aggregation, reduce inflammation and improve blood flow. From omega 6 fats are manufactured series 1 and series 2 prostaglandins. Like series 3 prostaglandins, series 1 prostaglandins are beneficial. On the other hand, series 2 prostaglandins promote inflammation and increase platelet aggregation.

This is why it is important to balance the amounts of omega 3 and omega 6 fats in the diet- aiming for a higher proportion of omega-3 fats.

Polyunsaturated oils are extremely susceptible to damage from heat, light, and oxygen. When exposed to these elements for too long, the fatty acids in the oil become oxidized. The oil becomes rancid which means it tastes and smells different. Oxidation also means free radicals. Free radicals are not a good thing – contributing to the development of degenerative diseases and cancer.

Hence, polyunsaturated oils should be stored in dark glass, tightly closed containers in a cool place. Also, cooking with oils high in polyunsaturates produces free radicals. A better choice for cooking are oils rich in monounsaturates (such as olive oil) which do not change in composition as much when heated. Saturated fats (like butter) also do not oxidize much when cooking, but only should be used in limited amounts.

If you want to increase your omega-3 intake, the foods providing the best omega-3 profiles are flaxseeds, walnuts and salmon. There are many other foods rich in omega-3 fats as well as the oils derived from these foods. A simple web search for "foods rich in omega-3 fats" will give you all kinds of information on this topic.

To your health!

# Rising Blood Sugar
# and Pre-Diabetes

I don't usually like to talk about myself. Ok, that's a lie. But, I recently had an experience with my own health that I thought might be of interest.

Like most folks, every year or so I go to the doctor for a check-up. So a couple of weeks back I fasted for 12 hours and went early in the morning for my blood work. Not fun. The test isn't bad, but I am grumpy without coffee in the morning.

The doctor gave me a shopping list of tests that I can have and I chose. It's the most comprehensive set of tests I have ever had and the results of them were quite enlightening.

Here's some background. I am a 48 year old, pre-menopausal woman, slim build, very physically active and lifetime vegetarian (ovo-lacto). A doctor's dream patient.

As you might expect, my cholesterol readings have always been great – which is to be expected for a fit pre-menopausal woman (estrogen has beneficial effects on cholesterol). However, a few years ago, my tests showed that my blood sugar readings were "high", with normal hovering around 100 mg/dl (5.5 mmol/L).

Readings were "high", with normal I was shocked and concerned that I was on the verge of developing pre-diabetes. The second year, the same test results. I got used to the idea that I was likely to develop Type II diabetes in 10 years. After all, for 20+ years I had been doing all the "right" things according to the American Diabetes Association guidelines – yet the numbers were inching higher.

I began to read bunches on pre-diabetes and what to expect. From reading, I knew that scientists are beginning to find more and more connections between not only high blood sugar and heart disease, but also links between blood sugar and pancreatic, colon, breast, prostate, and other cancers. I started to research ways to help myself nutritionally and fitness-wise. After a lot of research from traditional medicine to alternative, fitness and nutrition, I developed a plan and followed it for a year and a half.

To see if the plan is working, in the recent check-up, I asked for the full blood sugar testing including the test that measures blood sugar ranges over a 3 month period. When the tests came back, my blood sugar was 80 and stable over 3 months. My cholesterol profile was even better than previous years. Great!

Then, I compared the recent test with medical records kept over the last 20 years. I saw something amazing...my blood sugar, cholesterol and other readings (liver function etc.) are the same now as they were in 1991 – when I was 32 years old.

After that time, the readings slowly increased. By 1996, my blood sugar reading was 100. Why wasn't this pointed out at the time? Well, back in 1996 the "normal" ranges for blood sugar were between 70 and 140. So, 100 was well within range.

The designated normal ranges have dropped significantly in the last few years. Now we have intermediate ranges called pre-diabetes. (110-125) This is used largely as an intervention technique, because if caught at these early stages, half of people will not develop diabetes if they change their habits and lifestyle.

So, back to my story: what was the plan I developed? What did I change over the last year and a half that so significantly lowered blood sugar readings?

Here's what I did:

- Reduced dramatically the bread, pasta, rice and other grain-based things, brown or white, to less than once per week.

- Rarely ate sugar – paying specific attention to hidden sugars in food. No fruit juice or sports drinks

- Ate many more vegetables and raw vegetables. Used fruit in moderation.

- Added lots more protein foods: beans, nuts, lean dairy, eggs, soy (a non-vegetarian would include meat/poultry/fish)

- Had 5 to 6 small meals per day rather than 3 big ones.

- Added cinnamon daily.

- Included chromium and magnesium to my daily vitamin intake (multi-vitamin, antioxidants and essential fatty acids)

- Added more weight training to my workout.

- Practiced conscious stress reduction techniques

Since I did not approach the problem of lowering my blood sugar using the scientific method, it's impossible to say which of the above items individually helped lower the sugar readings. Put all together, they did work...dramatically.

So if you or anyone you know has blood sugar increases, it's worth giving the things above a try. At the very least, you will be following a sound nutrition, fitness and wellness plan which certainly is good for you!

# It's Not Just What You Eat, It's How You Cook It

If you are really serious about healthy nutrition, it's time to reconsider not just what you are eating, but also how you are cooking the food. More and more studies are showing that grilling, frying and broiling (especially flame-broiling) meat products produces toxins known as Advanced Glycation End-Products, known as AGEs. The highest amounts of these toxins are found in fried chicken and broiled or grilled meats.

So what?

Here's what… AGEs accumulate in the body over time. Older people naturally have higher levels than younger ones, but when a younger person eats a diet high in these compounds they too have high levels.

A new study at Mount Sinai School of Medicine that supports a previous study by the National Institute on Aging found that the levels of AGEs in a person's body were determined by direct dietary intake of them rather than the number of calories, fats or sugars they ingest.

In other words, eating fried, grilled and broiled meats raises the levels of AGEs.

AGEs were previously known to be associated with diabetes and insulin imbalance; but there's more. High levels of AGE's cause oxidative damage which increases inflammatory processes and inhibits synthesis of nitric oxide.

Nitric oxide is needed by many systems in the body including the cardiovascular system, immune system, nervous system and the brain.

Inflammation is the underlying cause for a bunch of diseases including heart disease, kidney damage and Alzheimer's disease. Basically, AGEs increase the body's inflammatory processes – and hence aging.

Too many AGEs in the body begin to overwhelm the ability of the body to get rid of these toxins and so they accumulate. The researchers found that people aged 65 and older had 35% more accumulated AGEs than those under age 45. The speculation is that the kidneys loose efficiency as we get older and are unable to clear the AGEs as efficiently as a younger person.

You have probably heard a lot about trans fats in the last few years. Well, the researchers in this study are advocating the same sort of approach with AGEs: that people eat less fried, grilled or broiled meat and that food nutrition labels reflect the AGE's in the products. They advocate cooking methods that keep the water content of the meat higher.

Boiling, stewing and poaching meats avoids production of AGEs.

Since those cooking methods also are lower in fat calories, cooking that way will make us thinner, healthier and younger! Not bad.

# BODY

# Mirror, Mirror on the Wall...

Body image is a topic that usually makes one think of teenaged girls starving themselves thin. But most people, no matter how old or young, have a feeling or image of the way their body should look. This image is composed of the actual view in the mirror combined with life experience, such as the image of our own younger/fitter/slimmer body, and the expectations of the way their body "should" look. This "should" comes from media images, parental influences, peers, past experiences or who knows what....

In my many years of fitness training I have noticed one common pattern among new fitness participants. Most newbies start a fitness program to "get healthy and fit" and to change a particular body part. Note the operative phrase here is particular body part. For example, it's common for men to want to lose the fat roll around the mid section ("love handles") and for women want to trim the hips.

Have you ever really observed other people in your gym? If you do, you will notice that there are a lot of men doing upper body and arm work and a lot of women doing lower body work. I recently prescribed outer and inner thigh (abductor/adductor) work to a client who was an experienced body builder. Yet he had never trained these muscles specifically because he felt these exercises "were for women"!

Yes, we've all heard for years that it's impossible to "spot reduce" by exercising the body part, but emotionally this idea is hard to own...especially for newbies. I can't tell you how many times I have given a person a weight training and aerobics style fitness program which is enthusiastically started but at the 1 month follow up it's revealed that the exerciser has thrown out exercises that did not target the imagined problem area and replaced them with extra sets of the exercises that did.

Now, take that same newbie, get him or her working out regularly and systematically for about 6 months and you get the beginnings of real body transformation. What does this mean? It means different things to different people, but to me it means BALANCE...and balance is beautiful. A body system that is in balance moves better, stands straighter (this means looking better in your clothes), can be trusted to perform physical activities longer and better and is less likely to sustain injury. Yes, the person's perceived "problem areas" change, but so do all the non-problem areas.

The most interesting thing that I've noticed is that with this body change, the newbie who is now truly enthusiastic about his or her changed body also has redefined goals and expectations of what it means to transform their body...and what a healthy body should look like. It's very common to hear women clients say that they had no idea that their arms could be so attractive and shapely and for men to comment that they like having legs that aren't so "skinny". These very same women started out avoiding arm work because they only were thinking about slimmer hips.

After six months or so when new trainees start to see real differences, they talk about how they feel a real sense of accomplishment (it is hard work to get there no doubt about it!). They begin to formulate new fitness goals which are surprisingly different than the ones they started with. These folks have not only begun to transform their bodies, they have transformed their thinking. Their perception of their body, or body image, has become very different.

They KNOW they look good and feel good!

# Wisdom Through the Ages

I have a friend who is much older than she looks. Since I know that she generally takes good care of herself by eating well and exercising (great skin and what a fit body!), I once asked her if there was one thing she did that she felt contributed the most to her youthful look and she replied "I try to sleep long enough every night so that I wake up naturally". (I had hoped to get the name of some new amazing beauty treatment).

There's lots of new research out there attempting to fully understand the effect that disturbed sleep has on health. Although, those of us who have had a newborn baby in the house KNOW without the science what sleep deprivation does to you...OH BOY!

But seriously, there are more and more indicators of the association between lack of sleep and many of the "big" killers.

Lack of sleep appears to increase the production of stress hormones and driving up blood pressure - a major risk factor for heart attacks and strokes. Moreover, people who are sleep-deprived have higher levels of chemicals in the blood which indicate a heightened state of inflammation in the body, a risk factor for heart disease, stroke, cancer and diabetes (big killers).... All of which can lead to a shortened life.

Scientists tell us that, for the majority of people, seven to nine hours per night of sleep is needed for optimal functioning. And as more and more studies of the body processes that take place during sleep are uncovered, it becomes clearer that getting enough sleep is really important in the prevention of disease. The research even points to the idea that, in addition to the big killers, the risk of obesity increases with less than 6 or 7 hours of sleep per night. Obesity? Really?

Hold on. The idea that excess fat accumulation happens because of lack of sleep goes against my personal logic. After all, if you stay awake more hours it seems like you would burn more calories than if you were sleeping. Well, apparently you do burn more calories....but there's a pitfall: the brain chemicals involved with appetite signals go wacky. So much for that line of thinking...

The two recently identified chemicals involved with appetite are called leptin and ghrelin. Leptin, which is produced by the fat cells, suppresses appetite and ghrelin increases it. When the duration of the sleep is shorter or sleep is interrupted, the leptin levels drop and ghrelin increases, and sends hunger signals to the brain. That explains the popularity of the midnight snack!

Back to my friend's idea of sleeping until you wake up naturally. Last summer, I decided to try it for a couple of weeks (with the alarm set as backup in case I slept TOO late). To do this, I had to go to bed a bit earlier. You know what happened? Except for the one night I stayed up too late with my girlfriends and woke up too early, I slept between seven and eight hours. I felt great and looked rested. More importantly, I became more tuned into my own body's sleep requirements. Good lesson.

The gist of it all? My friend is on to something. Sleep IS...good for you.

# Combating the Effects of a Desk Job

As you might already recognize from my previous chapter, I am a crusader for correcting muscle imbalances. Muscle imbalances occur in all of us through daily activities and movements. In this chapter, I would like to discuss the types of imbalances that occur in people who sit for long periods of time, say in a computer-related job or taxi driver.

If you are reading this now, you are probably in a sitting position (unless you are in a Starbucks at one of the standing internet stations, and also having a coffee YUM). Focus on your body position. What muscles do you feel are shorter and which are longer (contracted vs stretched)? Basically, the muscles of the front of your body are shorter and the back side are longer. If you are using your mouse or typing, your shoulders and neck are rounded a bit forward.

Ok, so the muscles of your chest, abdomen and hip flexors (connect top of legs to torso in front) are tighter, and your butt and back (especially upper back) are looser. Over time, this position weakens the muscles of the back, butt and back of the upper leg and leaves the body with over tight hip flexors (putting stress on the low back) and tight chest muscles (pulling shoulders forward). A rounded spine is not good either!

"That's ok", you say. "I go to the gym and do strength training"….great!!! BUT I think you can see where I am going with this…

If you are sitting at a computer or driving a car (or any other sitting activity) for long periods of time, it's a good idea to emphasize working out the backside of your body a bit more than the front. In other words, build the muscles of your lower, middle and upper back, the gluteal muscles (derrière) and the back of your upper leg. Stretch a bit more those muscles of the front like the quadriceps (front of the upper leg), hip flexors (front of the pelvic bones) and pectorals (chest).

To illustrate this further, stand up from your desk and arch your back. Drop your head back and let your arms fall down and back. Basically, this is the opposite position from sitting.  How does that feel?  I bet your back and shoulders say AAAHHH, good.  In this position, the muscles of your back side are shortened and the front ones are lengthened.

In yoga, there are many poses that involve arching the back.  Even the ancient masters knew about stretching and building opposing muscle groups to achieve "body balance"!

Taking this idea one step further.... In the gym or in your regular exercise routine, strengthen the muscles of your back, derrière and back of upper leg and you will see and feel the difference in your posture, with less back, shoulder and neck aches from your job.

For advice on which exercises build these muscle groups, talk to your trainer or check out the many books on the subject.

# Is It Just a Mid Life Crisis?

How often have you heard someone say "It's just a mid-life crisis"?

Nowadays, the terms mid-life crisis and male menopause seem to be popular explanations for odd behaviors exhibited by the men over 40. Are they the same thing? And what in the world is andropause?

Admittedly, there does seem to be a number of men who begin to act strangely in their 40s and 50s. Many a Hollywood movie has been based on this theme for sure.

I experienced this with my ex-husband of many years. It started insidiously. Sometime after he turned 40, I started noticing some attitude and behavior changes.

First, he started questioning whether to change a job which he always had enjoyed before. Over the next few years he began to exercise MUCH more, seemed preoccupied, irritable and more competitive. Then, it accelerated with strange manners of dress, excessive drinking, bar hopping, infidelity and finally leaving the family.

Was it just marital unhappiness, general midlife funk, depression and/or hormonal changes that caused this? Could it really be hormonal?

What are the scientists saying?

More and more the medical community and men themselves are acknowledging that something is going on. Research shows us that men do experience hormonal changes starting in midlife which include gradual loss of testosterone, DHEA, HGH and adrenal hormones, an increase in the proteins that bind to testosterone (making it unavailable) and aromatase which converts testosterone to estrogen.

Unlike women, where menopausal changes are pretty abrupt, men's changes happen over a period of years generally between the ages of 40 and 55. The effects and symptoms are hard to quantify because they are psychological in addition to physiological. Often evidence is anecdotal: men report feeling different.

There is a wide variation in the changes in healthy men so the symptoms will range from very little to extreme enough to use hormone replacement therapy.

Some of the typically reported conditions related to reductions in androgens (male hormones) are:

- Low sex drive

- Emotional, psychological and behavioral changes

- Decreased muscle mass

- Loss of muscle strength

- Increased upper and central body fat

- Osteoporosis or weak bones and back pain

- Cardiovascular risk

Now, earlier I discussed that as a man ages his body begins to convert more testosterone into estradiol (estrogen). Too much estrogen in a man's body is not a good thing because estrogen negates testosterone. So, some men with normal levels of testosterone will still have symptoms of andropause because the testosterone:estrogen ratios in the body are whacky.

What Can You Do About It?

1.  Stay Strong and Lean
    So how to keep testosterone high and estrogen low? Keep yourself strong and lean. Why? Fat cells contain aromatase – the guys that convert testosterone to estrogen. More fat cells = more estrogen. This is true for women too!
    Building and maintaining muscle mass requires free testosterone, so building and maintaining muscle mass trains the body to use testosterone efficiently.
    So, the idea behind slowing down the effects of diminishing testosterone would be to increase or at least maintain muscle mass and bone density while keeping the heart strong and fat away.
    Hmmm, this looks like the goal of any good fitness and nutrition program. That's good news!

2. Watch What Goes Into Your Body
   Zinc, Alcohol and some Prescription Drugs.
   Zinc inhibits the actions of aromatase in the body. Getting adequate levels of zinc from the diet is important to keep estrogen levels down. Zinc is also important for the manufacture of testosterone by the body. Foods rich in zinc include meat, poultry, dairy, nuts, beans and whole grain foods.
   Alcohol drives estrogen levels up. Since the liver helps excrete hormones and chemicals from the body anything that diminishes liver function results in higher estrogen levels.
   Some prescription drugs can mess with hormone levels. It's a good idea to check this out with your doctor if you feel you are having some symptoms related to lowered testosterone.

3. Listen to Other People
   Men, if you are over 40, and a family member or friend says that you are acting out of character, talk to your doctor about it. It might not be "her hormones"….it might be YOURS!!

# Sports Injury: Making Lemons into Lemonade

**M**y sister died yesterday. She would have been 55 years young next week. She fell down a flight of stairs and hit her head. Just like that – gone. Over the last five years, she battled breast cancer, marital separation after 32 years and her daughter leaving home for university (the last one is both happy and sad for her). She had just begun the journey of her second adulthood, a new adventure and a new life.

When something like this happens, it really highlights the element of uncertainty that pervades our lives. Many of us go through the day comfortable in our routines and never think about the external forces that could change those routines forever....until something happens to create change.

Living through adversity is hard at first, but if we are aware of the ways in which we grow and change, what is learned by living the hardship turns out to be more precious than that which was lost.

Is this a fitness chapter? Of course it is!

Have you ever had an injury that kept you from your fitness activity for a period of time? What did you do?

Well, primarily you were followed your doctor's advice (which is usually to rest for a period of time), right??!! Of course you did.... But then what?

There are several alternatives to choose from when recovering from an injury. It comes down to mindset – are you going to let this injury defeat you, set you back slightly or are you going to use the recovery to grow and develop your fitness in other ways?

Here are some examples:

- **Defeat:** "I am getting too old to do this activity". "I get hurt whenever I do this activity". "I better do something more gentle".

- **Setback:** "It's only an injury. After I recover I will begin again". "I need to find less risky ways to do this activity".

- **Opportunity:** "I can't participate in the activity during recovery, but I can spend the time learning more about the activity so as to get better at it". "I can ask my doctor and fitness trainer if there are some complementary activities that I can do while I am recovering from this injury" (eg,, swimming if it's a leg injury).

Often, an injury can lead us to do activities that we never thought to do before. I once ran a marathon with a lady who ripped her Achilles tendon halfway through training. It was her first marathon and she had her heart set on finishing what she started. Her doctor told her that she would recover in time to do the marathon if she was careful. However, she would not have time to train properly after recovery. At first, she thought she had to quit.

I suggested to her that she "run" in the swimming pool to keep her fitness level up while her leg was recovering. What I didn't recognize at first was that her recovery time was going to be long enough that she would end up water running right up to the week before the marathon. She literally spent 4 hours in the swimming pool a couple of times before the marathon! (We organized a group of friends who were assigned times to be at the pool with her and help cheer her on).

She finished the marathon strong and without injury! As the saying goes, she took a lemon and made lemonade. What an inspiration...

What else came out of the experience? She began to enjoy swimming for fitness and continued to swim after the marathon in addition to running. She went on to compete in triathlons.

So, the next time you are faced with a fitness or sports injury, think.....
LEMONADE!

# Body is Beautiful

Do you have moments where you say "WOW! Life is truly wonderful!"?

This morning started out as most others. I was having my workout. My child left for school and my husband spent a few minutes entertaining me (he is a funny guy), before leaving for his workplace. As I started moving to the music, this sudden feeling of joy and thankfulness came over me like a warm blanket. A truly inspiring moment of great awareness.

After finishing the morning workout, I surfed the web for forums on gratitude to see what people were talking about. Many of the writings were about being thankful for what we do have rather than focusing on what we don't as an important feature of optimism and success. There was one particularly interesting discussion on being thankful for our bodies and what the body can do.

Spiritual leaders and psychologists alike tell us that "gratitude" is a very important part of emotional health, spiritual wellness and good relationships. As kids, we learn to thank people for doing nice things for us and we learn about being thankful for the material things, people, victories, challenges and situations that we have.

I was very lucky to have a father who was always optimistic – a big part of which came from his deeply rooted feelings of gratefulness for all aspects of his life. From him I learned to grow and change with each challenge and be thankful for the opportunity to do so. He always said that everything happens because fate is working to take us to where we need to be.

Optimism and gratitude are not only components of emotional and spiritual wellness, but also physical wellness and hence…fitness. An easy demonstration of this is the person who survives cancer. Often it's the attitude of "I am sure that I will beat this and in the meantime I will be thankful for everyday" that determines this person's survival. If you have ever been close to someone in this situation, you understand when I say how wonderful these folks are to be around – the attitude is contagious! Think Lance Armstrong.

A few years back I lost optimism for a time. My ex-husband of over 15 years left me for someone else after having a long term affair. I cried everyday for nearly a year and started to be afraid that I would always be sad. As time went by, my health deteriorated. I couldn't eat, lost muscle weight, couldn't sleep etc.

My medical exam tests that year showed that this pessimism was in fact affecting my health. It was only when I was able to stop focusing on loss and recognize what I had gained from the experience did my health improve. Also, I was able to open myself to the idea of "dating" (dating after 20 years is quite exciting!). Eventually dating led me to meet the funny guy from the first paragraph and many other new adventures!

When you are exercising, or just going about your daily routine, do you stop and marvel at the beauty and functionality of your own body? Or do you focus on what's wrong with it either aesthetically or mechanically? The body is an incredible piece of work. Each body is unique. Your body houses "you", transports you and gives you the ability to feel, see, hear and communicate among other things. It's truly something to be thankful for.

Appreciation of your body is key to keeping it healthy. Focusing on what your body can do will allow you to build fitness and stay positive even when your workouts (or daily life) become particularly challenging.

Always be thankful for your BEAUTIFUL body that serves you so well!

# MIND

# Are We Having Fun Yet?

Like taxes, stress is a part of everyone's life. The "experts" tell us that some stress is good because without it there would be no motivation to do anything! However, if you are like me, serious stress and anxiety makes me feel bad physically – I am unable to eat. This can't be good!

For most of us, stress is low-level most of the time. Our daily tasks and relationships give us a bit of stress but not major anxiety. The body's response to low-level stressors is designed to motivate us to action with a slightly raised heart rate and increased mental clarity –similar to the response to caffeine.

In times where stress levels go higher, the responses are what many people call the "fight or flight" response. The body sends blood to the extremities to get ready for action! These responses are normal and good for you – except when the stress levels remain high for a long time. When the body perpetually stays in a stressed state, the systems begin to break down. Think of it like a car engine where the throttle is stuck and the engine is constantly "revved up". Not only will it consume A LOT of gasoline, but the mechanical parts will wear out faster.

So what to do to protect ourselves from this? RELAX of course....and EXERCISE. Exercise helps us relax both physiologically and, if it's enjoyable, provides a mental escape from the stressor. The physiological effects of exercise include release of morphine-like chemicals (which include beta-endorphins) that give us a sense of well-being. Have you ever heard the term Runner's High? This is caused by the release of "endorphins" into the blood. Since these chemicals stay in the blood for several hours after stopping the activity, the "feel good" feeling remains for a while.

OK, so we know why exercise can help with anxiety and stress. But what are some of the ways regular exercise keeps us healthy in normal, low-level stress, times?

Here's some from the top of my head:

- Using a daily dose of natural "feel good" chemicals is better than drugs or alcohol!!

- Looking fit, healthy and strong (It's ok to admit that looking good makes you feel good!)

- Feeling good from accomplishment and improvement.

- Escaping from the daily grind for an hour – change of scene.

- Keeping the body systems prepared to handle high-level stress.

The key to lowering stress with exercise is that you **ENJOY** the exercise that you choose to do. If you hate going to the gym, it's not going to lower your stress – in fact it probably will add some! Also, studies are showing over and over that even low intensity exercise helps anxiety, so any activity you enjoy is good. For me, when I am under stress, nothing works better than a good sweaty dance session. The music, movement and high heart rate just melt away my troubles. Some of my clients even tell me that the sense of achievement from competitive sports makes them feel less stressed!

The bottom line? To decrease the effects of stress on your body, pick a fitness or sports activity you enjoy, do it regularly and **HAVE FUN**.

# What's Right for Aunt Sally Might Not Be Right for You

If you have ever been through hard times (haven't we all), you were probably given advice by so many different people. For many life situations, there often seems to be as many opinions as people giving advice!

We are all products of our experiences. Emotions and judgments are really the result of "where we were when". The values we were taught as kids, the life experiences that we have had as well as current situations all come together to form our perceptions of reality.

Fitness and nutrition are no exceptions. Take any cross section of people, say 100, and ask their opinion on a particular fitness idea, and you will probably get 100 different opinions. This is the dilemma I see often with clients. Many, before I see them, have spent a period of time "trying out" this diet or that workout plan because it worked for their friend or their sister gave it to them and so on.

My favorite example of this is my spouse used to be asked for fitness advice because he was fit and married to a fitness instructor! He had some good ideas. He knew what worked…. for HIM.

What works for one person may not work for another. Why? Physiologically, the science is pretty much the same. For optimum fitness and health, we all need a combination of resistance exercise (muscles and bones), aerobic exercise (cardio-vascular, lungs), stretching (joint health), good nutrition (fuel) and enough sleep (rebuild). The trick of all this is the how to get these things and enjoy it….because enjoyment leads to motivation.

Let's say that Aunt Sally walks with a group 4 miles, 3 times per week. She eats a healthy diet of lean protein, veggies and fruit and goes to yoga class 2 times per week. She loves her "program", which works for her because she loves it. Aunt

Sally gets a lot of social time from her workouts, which keeps her going. The time she spends is more valuable to her than just fitness. She rarely misses her sessions.

Aunt Sally eventually convinces her niece Elizabeth, who thinks fitness is a necessary evil, to join her. Elizabeth begins with enthusiasm, but after a month she doesn't feel like she is getting results and starts missing sessions. Why?

If we asked Elizabeth, she would probably say that fitness is "just not her thing and she doesn't enjoy it". But, maybe Elizabeth hasn't found the activities that give her what she really needs beyond fitness. In this case, Aunt Sally meant well, but her "mentoring" was actually counterproductive to Elizabeth's fitness success. Elizabeth has now reinforced her feeling that she doesn't like physical activity.

The same thing holds with "diets" (I personally don't like the term). Let's bring up Aunt Sally again. One day Elizabeth, who now thinks that a diet is what she needs since exercise is out, asks Aunt Sally if she could help her lose weight with a diet. Aunt Sally gives her the diet book that got her started on the road to healthy eating.

When Aunt Sally read the book, she knew that the diet was very strict with types of food and timing of meals. For her, it was great to have a structure to follow. It was all so organized, as she liked all things in her life.

Elizabeth, on the other hand, tried to follow the diet exactly as recommended. Within a few days, she was very frustrated because she felt that dieting is just too difficult and inflexible. She decided that dieting doesn't work and she just needs to "cut way back" on the amount of food she was eating. This is good – except that most of the food she is eating is nutritionally empty to begin with! Now she's hungry and inadequately nourished.

Elizabeth would be better served by learning about and following sound nutritional principles rather than following a rigid diet plan. It's just not her style.

Are you having trouble starting or sticking with your fitness plan? Here's an approach to get you thinking....

1. Look inside.

   What drives you? What makes you happy? Why do you want to be fit? Why do you want to eat right? What activities do you enjoy doing (both physical activities and other hobbies)? Are you a social person or do you prefer to be alone? What are the limiting factors in your lifestyle? How much time do you want to devote to fitness? What type of job do you have? Do you like changing your activities often or do you prefer a more predictable routine?

2.  Look outside.
    What resources are available?  Do you have sports activities you
    might enjoy available?  Is there a gym close by?  Is there a dance
    studio close by?  Are there organized events like fun runs you
    could train for?  Can you find books on the subject of fitness and
    nutrition?  Do you know any fitness trainers or coaches?

3.  Put it together.
    A good fitness plan includes the elements of: muscle strength,
    joint flexibility, aerobic (heart, lungs) training, sound nutrition
    and rest.  So, pick out the activities available to you that you like
    and see if the combination gives you all the elements in this list.

Elizabeth, when she goes through this process, is surprised to figure out that
there are some fitness activities available she would enjoy.  She knows she is social,
wants to keep generally fit and healthy, has time after work, needs organized activities and likes variety (why Aunt Sally's program didn't appeal to her).

Elizabeth's program looks like this:

1 day per week, join a football (soccer) league (aerobic)
1 day per week, yoga class or Tai Chi (flexibility, muscle, mental focus)
1 day per week salsa dancing class (aerobic)
1 day weight training (muscle)
Some weeks: social dancing on the weekends (aerobic, relaxation)
She's got a good plan..... FOR HER!

# Lessons from a Boomerang

R esilience: What does that word mean to you?
    To me, it means learning from mistakes and using that knowledge to create positive change. Being resilient in the face of adversity requires that a person be honest enough with him or herself to see their own mistakes for what they are without blame (self or others), reflect on what could have been done differently and have the courage to try again. Resilience involves taking the "if only...." statement and transforming it into "next time…"

Recently, I came across a statement published in the American Journal of Clinical nutrition that said 90% of successful dieters had failed before with many of the dieters reporting several gains and losses before achieving their goals. By itself, the statement is pretty uninformative, but it does say one thing: the successful dieters didn't give up. In fact, I would venture to speculate that most of these people kept trying different things, learning with each failure what worked and what didn't until they found what worked for them.

It has been my observation that the same thing is true for exercise and fitness. What's the difference between a really fit person and one that isn't? The fit person doesn't let failures like choosing a fitness program that they don't like or otherwise doesn't work for them stop them. They take the knowledge gained from their mistakes and use it to move forward.

Isn't this how champions are made?

Can a couch potato become a champion athlete? Of course! It takes more than just the intention to do it, though. It takes commitment and a mindset change. It takes being honest with yourself about your motives. It means releasing your fear of change, fear of failure, fear of success and dependence on other people's opinions of your choices. It involves looking at past attempts and reflecting on both the good and the bad about those attempts without judging yourself negatively.

Let's use an example of a fictional person named Roger. Roger is a successful scientist and has a lovely family. He's happily married, has three children and all the "trappings" related to his success. Life's good. He has one thing in his life that bothers him: his health. When he turned 38, he started to show medical signs of years of inactivity and overweight – high cholesterol. At age 40, he knows he needs to do something to improve his health, but the motivation isn't stronger than the "pain" of changing his lifestyle....yet.

Over the years, Roger has sporadically gone to the gym and not eaten too much "junk" food but he has never been particularly motivated. He chose to be too busy to make his own health a priority. Whenever he starts a new fitness program and gets frustrated he feels like a failure. Failure is very a very uncomfortable feeling for Roger. He doesn't like it, so he runs from it.

Wham! One day he has a mild heart attack and ends up in the hospital. The pain of change just became less important than his motivation to be healthy! Roger must change his life or lose it. BIG motivator. Sadly, this type of earth shaking experience is all too often the impetus for change.

Roger no longer has trouble with mindset changes when faced with the alternative which is possibly premature death. But what about our second fictional person, Elizabeth?

Elizabeth is 35, has a successful career, great family and no health problems. She has always felt healthy and is mildly active. She intends to work out 4 hours per week but usually only manages on average two hours per week. She is always "dieting", going from one fad diet to the other. She feels like she has 3 kilos (6.6 pounds) too much weight. Not enough to impact her health.

So, what really are her honest motives to change? Does she have any? When she is honest with herself she knows she is motivated by the way her body looks. This makes her uncomfortable because she feels that other people would think she is vain or superficial (I am sure that her husband doesn't mind one bit that she wants to look good!). This uncomfortable feeling is keeping her from changing her mindset and developing strategies for success. All because of other people's opinions about what should or should not be important to her.

See why it's important for Elizabeth to reflect on her fears and impediments to fitness success? It's also important for her to come to terms with the idea that what she has been doing hasn't accomplished what she wants it to. Then, she will need to identify and embrace changes that she decides will work for her. This self-reflection will lead her down her own personal championship road.

Real lasting change comes from resiliency… growing from our mistakes. Champions are made one mistake at a time! Like a boomerang, they always come back for more.

# Are You Fit...Emotionally?

This week, I was surfing the web for ideas for fitness articles and something really caught my attention. It was an article on emotional fitness by Dr. Mathew Anderson called "Fat and Emotional Fitness".

What is emotional fitness? Well, it's really about our ability to recognize what each of our emotions are telling us, as well as being comfortable with all of our emotions and those of others. Dr. Anderson's premise is that emotional fitness is an important factor in weight control because so many of us eat, not only when we are hungry, but also when we do not recognize our emotions for what they are.

The following "checklist" is excerpted from "Fat and Emotional Fitness":
An Emotionally Fit Person...

- Knows how she/he feels at any given moment and can give that feeling a name. Such as angry, sad, happy, frustrated, joyful, excited, afraid and hurt.

- Can and does communicate those feelings to at least one other person daily.

- Can "be with" her/his intense feelings without having to act them out. To act out means to allow the feeling to dictate emotion driven action such as overeating or any addictive behavior, striking out at others or becoming self-destructive.

- Understands that emotions, including intense emotions, are a normal part of life.

- Does not make any emotion a forbidden emotion, even sexual feelings, sadness, fear and anger.

- Can hear, accept and "be with" the emotions of others, even if they are sometimes intense, without judging them.

- Understands that emotions, properly experienced, accepted and managed, contribute to one's quality of life.

- Understands that chronic, extremely intense emotions are related to past wounds and traumas and need attention and deeper exploration, possibly with a professional. The very emotionally fit person will get the help she/he needs.

From Dr. Anderson's list, I can see that not being "in tune" with one's emotions would cause all kinds of unsavory behaviors and overeating can be very self-destructive. What about taking this idea to other addictive or self -destructive behaviors – in particular exercise addiction?

Like overeating, over exercising is a socially accepted addiction. In other words, on the surface it appears to be a good thing. Also, it seems like only the person engaged in the behavior is affected by it. However, if you have ever been involved with someone with an addiction or self-destructive behavior of any kind, you know that friends, family members and work colleagues are all affected in one way or the other.

Exercise addiction is no exception. Exercise requires time and energy and when it becomes excessive, not only does the addict get hurt a lot, but the time and energy needed to sustain important relationships also goes to exercise. But exercise is good, right! YES – unless it takes control over your life. Even professional athletes and fitness trainers know when to stop.

How do you know if you are over exercising? Well, probably the best indicator is if close family members or friends are REALLY complaining about how much time you are spending at it. Things like, "Is it really so important that you spend 4 hours per day at the gym?" will be said. If you really don't feel like exercising because you are so tired yet you feel compelled to work out anyway, could be a sign – especially if you do this often. If you insist on exercising when you are sick or injured and have been told by your doctor to rest, this too could be a sign of addiction.

If you are over exercising or engaging in any behavior that is causing relationship problems, work problems or serious stress, try looking inward to understand what your feelings really are telling you. Emotional fitness is just as important as physical and mental fitness for keeping us free from illness and injury. Your body depends on it!

# Type D Personality?

We have all heard of Type A personality types, but have you heard about Type D, or distress, personality? There was an observation made by, Johan Denollet, a Belgian psychologist, of cardiac patients a while back. Denollet noticed that some patients with extensive cardiac problems were optimistic and went through rehabilitation enthusiastically, while others, who had only mild problems were more pessimistic and did not follow rehabilitation activities well. Denollet was interested in the why of this. Out of his work came a 14 question survey designed to determine whether a person has something he termed "distress" personality.

His survey identifies overall stress in terms of states of "negative affectivity" (worry, irritability and gloom) and social inhibition (reticence and social inhibition) and it has been surprisingly helpful in predicting cardiovascular health – in particular hypertension and coronary heart disease. Those studied who had existing heart disease and high distress scores were less responsive to treatment and were more likely to die prematurely.

This idea of psychosocial factors playing a role in illness is not new, but it is finding its way more and more into mainstream health habits and healthcare. Since the advent of stress management for Type A personality types in prevention and treatment of heart disease, researchers are searching for other ways that stress and emotions affect our health.

One particularly interesting idea is that if depression and anger can increase our susceptibility to heart disease, what effect do positive emotions have on our health? One researcher showed that optimistic outlooks slow atherosclerosis in post menopausal women. Other researchers found that watching a funny movie for 15 minutes (hearty laughter) increases blood flow - similar to 45 minutes of aerobic exercise.

Gratitude is the topic of one study of people with neuromuscular disease. The results in a nutshell of interviewing these folks was that having a sense of gratitude increased the quality of their lives and lessened the rate of physical decline caused by their disease.

Dr. Dean Ornish, a heart disease expert and writer, states outright that love and intimacy (true connection) with others, or the lack of it, is at the root of what prevents and causes illness. He says: "I'm not aware of any other factor in medicine—not diet, not smoking, not exercise, not genetics, not drugs, not surgery—that has a greater impact on our quality of life, incidence of illness and premature death. In part, this is because people who are lonely are more likely to engage in self-destructive behaviors."

Dr. Ornish believes that a paradigm shift is needed in today's social makeup to guard our health. He believes that science is beginning to demonstrate that love, intimacy, compassion, forgiveness, community, altruism and service are very important to our health. He goes on to say that "being unselfish may be the most self-serving approach to life, for it helps free both the giver and recipient from suffering, disease, and premature death".

Isn't this what all of the world's philosophers, spiritual and religious leaders have been saying all along?

# Wellness and Making
# Good Choices

What do you think of when someone says the word wellness?  What does it mean to you?

Out of curiosity, I looked up "definition of wellness" on the web and a bunch of different results came up!  Many of them referred to being physically, medically or mentally well.

My favorite definition of wellness comes from the National Wellness Association of Singapore – "wellness is an active process of becoming aware of and making choices toward a more successful existence".  An active process….

To me, wellness represents the integration of physical, mental/emotional and spiritual fitness.  A healthy mind and a healthy body so to speak. Throughout our lives, all these components change constantly because of new experiences and learning along with the body changes…especially as we enter middle age and beyond.

Do you know anyone who in midlife has become depressed or suddenly changed their behavior to what seems like a crazy destruction of all aspects of their life?  We often refer to this sort of behavior as midlife crisis.  Everyone has changes in priorities, lifestyles etc. in midlife, but why do some seem to really go to extremes?

Psychologists tell us that very few people truly experience classic midlife crisis.  Most of the time, the most extreme cases of change either ends up being classic depression or the person has had chaotic interpersonal relationships/job loss etc.,  all their lives.

Perhaps, these people are just lacking the integrated components of wellness that I am referring to above.  In other words, they may get 1 or 2 components right, but just lose sight of the others. Something is missing…

For example, say John Anyman who is 40. He is very fit, goes to the gym, runs and is on his local soccer team. He has been married for 15 years, has an eight year old child and a profession that he enjoys (good job). But he walks around with the nagging feeling that something is missing in his life. He just can't decide what that is.

One day, John leaves his family, quits his job and moves to Morrocco to "find" himself. Five years later, John is no happier than he was before. Why? The nagging feeling that something is missing is still there. John changed the outward trappings of his life without turning inward. In addition, he now lives with the loss of his family and the guilt of hurting them.

Perhaps if John had looked at all the aspects of wellness, physical, mental, emotional and spiritual, seen which area was lacking in his life and made small changes first, he would have kept his family and gotten rid of the nagging feeling. To quote a common cliché: happiness begins within.

Many of us midlifers (me included) go through a sort of metamorphosis for a variety of reasons. In my case, this metamorphosis started because of family breakdown which lead me to reevaluate my life and set my own priorities of what is important. Unfortunately, I did not notice that something was missing for complete wellness before my life situation changed.

What had been missing for me? Emotional fitness. I had never before thought to define priorities in this area and therefore did not ask loved ones for what I needed. My emotions were left to be controlled by daily situations, and the behavior of my husband (who was having his own "midlife crisis") and child. I was on "autopilot" and feeling that my life was without love. It wasn't until my physical body started to show signs of my emotional pain, that I was able to see that there was something wrong in my approach to my life. Hence, my metamorphosis began…and continues! An active process…

The message here for fitness enthusiasts is that working out and eating right is only one part of what makes us healthy. If the balance is not there in the other areas of our lives, and we are not taking care of our emotional selves – our bodies will show the signs sooner or later.

Make good choices!

# Fitness as a Metaphor for Life

As I was reflecting the other day on my life up to now, it occurred to me that the process of getting fit is a metaphor for living a full life. Stay with me here....

To get fit one needs to 1) decide to do it, 2) decide how to do it (plan) 3) do it and 4) re-evaluate from time to time. It's simple – and is pretty much the way we conduct our lives in general. So let's look at this more closely.

Decide to Do It

Whatever you do, from improving your relationships, getting better at your job to getting fit, the first step is to decide to do it. But that by itself isn't always so easy. Why? Because wanting to do something isn't the same as doing it! How often have you heard "I was going to do that" or "if only I had more time?", you got the idea. Hope won't give you a strong heart or big muscles! Blaming others or life situations (not enough time, my wife won't let me, my dog ate my workout clothes, etc.) also won't increase muscle mass.

It's very common for fitness trainers to hear these sorts of comments after they explain to the client what needs to be done to get fit. It's hard work and many people "want" to be fit, but balk when they see the work involved.

It's the same with relationships. How many of us would have had children if we had known the time, energy and emotional commitment involved beforehand (be honest now!)? How many people get divorced because they just can't or don't spend the time, energy, emotional commitment and personal responsibility that's necessary for a fulfilling lifetime relationship? Or professional development...if getting a University degree were easy, everyone would do it!

Researchers say that if your parents were fit, you are more likely to follow a fitness lifestyle. People tend to be most comfortable with the patterns of behavior and communication styles learned from their parents. Psychologists say that even if your parents followed a very unhealthy lifestyle or had a terrible marriage, you are not doomed to make the same mistakes if you are aware of the behaviors and values that you learned from them that hold you back.

### Decide How to Do It

Ok, so you make a plan on how to get fit. Everyone does this differently. Some people research the web or get a book and follow it. Some people just join a sports team or some other activity that they like. Some people hire a professional trainer. All are good. All will increase fitness. Like any other plan, setting measurable goals helps not only to get motivated and focused but also for evaluation later.

Goal setting is something that most of us have learned to do in school and on our jobs, but I was really surprised when I went to a marriage counselor years ago who advised me to set some goals for my marriage as well. It was a valuable exercise because it made me look at what areas of my relationship were good for me, what areas I could improve on and what mistakes I had made that I didn't want to repeat. Also, it gave the counselor a platform to help me work on those areas of myself and hence my relationship(s). The same methodology is used by fitness trainers all the time.

### Do It

Well, Yea. Just do it....if you don't like it or it just doesn't work for you – try something else. Fitness, profession, family, health, skill development etc. all take a lifetime to do well. No pain, no gain as the saying goes. It's just plain old hard work.

### Re-evaluate

Learning from successes and mistakes is the key here. Just like your job or relationships, your body will change and so you will need to make changes. As you get fitter, you will be able to handle more intense workouts. If you get injured or develop illness, you will need to change your workouts to accommodate the injury.

And hence the metaphor argument: being flexible and willing to grow into our challenges serves us well in health, relationships, profession… and LIFE.

# Neuro-Linguistic Programming for Fitness?

Last week, an old friend of mine (who I have known for almost 30 years), was telling me about how he feels about the current state of his life. He used the term "empty contentment".

"Empty contentment". Wow, how do those words make you feel?

To me, the phrase is very emotionally provocative. So many feelings: sadness, wonder, sympathy… But here's a thought: the term evokes my emotions based on my own frame of reference and not my friend's. In other words, maybe for him feeling "empty contentment" with his life is good. For me, feeling "empty contentment" seems bad.

In the last year or so, there has been a lot of talk in self-help and wellness media about Neuro-Linguistic Programming (NLP). Have you heard of it? My reaction to my friend's comment led me to do some more reading on this topic. It's pretty interesting stuff.

A definition of NLP I came across is: "The common processes we experience to experience reality". In other words, reality is processed by our 5 senses and nervous system into experience. Our experience is then given meaning by language and non-verbal communication.

Basically, some researchers in the 1970s developed the idea based on earlier work by a family therapist, a gestalt therapist, an anthropologist and a hypnotist (interesting combination). The original study was to answer the question, "why do different people with the same education and opportunities achieve different levels of success?"

The researchers developed models of behaviors of successful people based on the interconnection between neurology, linguistics and patterns of behavior. Then, they used the models to see if a person's communication and behavior patterns can be re-programmed for success.

I first heard the term NLP when it started being used on athletes – which seems to be a pretty successful use for this sort of thing. Now, more and more, NLP is used to help previously unfit people develop a fitness mindset.

Going back the above premises behind NLP, that language and non-verbal communication gives meaning to our experience, it does make sense that if one is made aware of his or her own negative communication patterns, experience can be revised into more positive frames of reference. I would call it a "change of attitude".

For example, John Anyman left his family and moved to Morocco. Let's say that he wants to run a marathon but something stops him. His self talk is along the lines of "the training is too much and boring", "I might get hurt", "what if I don't do well on the day" etc. He wants to do it, but talks himself out of it. Perhaps NLP would help him go forward and succeed.

NLP is an interesting concept. As NLP has been used for a long time, there are tons of NLP practitioners and life coaches who can help you achieve your goals. If you are interested in finding out more, a web search or a bookstore is a good place to start.

# Words Do Hurt – Stop Bullying from Affecting Your Health

The man who quits his job because of harassment. The woman whose husband stays out late at night repeatedly and tells her he is entitled to do what he wants. The child whose parent tells him often "you are lazy".

What do these people have in common? All of them have relationships with bullies.

Bullies can be anywhere, at work, at school, on the road (road rage), in the mall or in the family.

When thinking about the term "bully", most people think of the kid on the playground who threatens to hit you if you don't give up your lunch money. This is your typical overt or garden variety of bully. When you were a kid, how did you feel about these bullies? Anxious? Afraid? Angry? Avoidant? Victimized?

What happens to the schoolyard bullies as adults? If they aren't in prison, they are in our workplace or on the street, basically anywhere. Most people around them recognize the negative behavior and they usually pay the price for it pretty fast. However, many of these folks have an undercurrent of hidden anger and hostility which puts them at greater risk for heart attack, stroke and self destructive behaviors.

Overt bullying is pretty easy to recognize because the body language and tone of voice is threatening (booming). Sentences like "You don't know what you are talking about" or "what's your problem?" are said. If a person is in a business meeting shouts out one of these sentences, attendees would be shocked, and think "wow, he or she seems angry. That behavior is not appropriate".

What about the more covert types of bullying? Covert bullying can be much more frightening, because it utilizes a vicious combination of verbal and emotional abuse. It's insidious. It's stressful. It's not obvious. It's confusing.

How do you recognize a bully when they aren't threatening to beat you up? Words, body language and just plain old trusting your feelings are key. All of us get angry from time to time, but bullies tend to ooze hostility much of the time. There is a tendency for them to believe that others have malicious intent towards them when they don't.

Covertly hostile people, on the other hand, leave you with nagging wonder. "Did I really do something wrong?" They display a public persona of a "nice guy" or "nice girl", so the targeted person is quite surprised when they are treated terribly – in private.

People who employ covert bullying tactics are adept at using deception to escape accountability – often blaming their accuser. If you, the targeted person try to fix the problem(s) you were accused of making, it doesn't seem to help. There is always something else that's wrong. Why?

The hostile person has decided to target YOU. This is part of the personality of the hostile person. Many don't even realize why they do it or why they target a particular person. It's up to them to recognize that their behavior is unacceptable and decide to stop.

Patricia Evans, the author of "The Verbally Abusive Relationship", "Controlling People" and others, says it is all about CONTROL. Evans notes that men are the majority of verbal abusers (sorry gentlemen); but the number of women seems to be increasing. She theorizes this is due to socialization: for centuries, men were given the cultural message of the "right" to dominate.

According to Evans, "verbal abuse is hurtful, it attacks the nature and abilities of the target, may be overt (angry outbursts, name calling, blaming, accusations) or covert (very subtle, like brainwashing), may be voiced in a concerned way, is manipulative and controlling, insidious, unpredictable, expresses a double message and it ESCALATES over time!"

The following is a list of categories with some examples that Evans sites in her book:

1. Withholding. "You never let me talk"
2. Countering. "You are wrong"
3. Discounting. "You don't know what you are talking about"
4. Disguised as Joke. "What else can you expect from a woman"
5. Blocking and Diverting. "You always have to be right"
6. Accusing and Blaming. "I have had it with your constant complaining"
7. Judging and Criticizing. "You are crazy"
8. Trivializing. "Your concerns are not important".
9. Undermining. "No one asked your opinion".
10. Threatening. "Do what I want or I'll leave you".

11. Name Calling. "Jerk".
12. Forgetting. "I never agreed to do that (when he/she did)".
13. Ordering. "Shut up".
14. Denial. "You have got to be crazy".
15. Abusive Anger = Violence.

Emotionally abusive tactics include, but aren't limited to, lying and deception, lack of consideration, humiliation, exclusion, abandonment, ignoring, incessant teasing and starting rumors.

Both covert and overt bullies have a great deal of difficulty in work life and interpersonal relationships. Even the covertly hostile person who seems like such a nice person will show tell tale signs like more than one divorce, few close friends, difficulty keeping a job or chaotic relationships of some sort.

The closer the target is to the bully (such as spouse) and the longer it goes on, the more damage can be done. Even if the target doesn't have physical injuries, over time he/she can develop symptoms of traumatic stress or become depressed requiring medical and psychological help. Long term stress and depression can lead to a whole host of physical ailments and self-destructive behaviors.

We tell our kid's when harassed by a playground bully to tell them to stop, run away, talk to an adult about it, stay away from the bully and stay with other people so that the bully can't catch you alone.

This seems to be good advice for adults too. If you are being emotionally or verbally harassed, tell them to stop it, leave and tell other people about it. If it's covert, the people you tell may seem at first to not believe ("they seem so nice."), but, after some thought, usually it dawns on them that they too had an encounter with this person that didn't feel "right".

In short, if you are harassed/bullied:
1. Say "Stop it!
2. Leave.
3. Tell someone.

**If you feel you are in physical danger – SCREAM! RUN! CALL the POLICE!**

If you have found yourself feeling bullied, YOU are not causing the problem. You are the current target. There's nothing you can do except leave. If you try to tell them what they are doing to themselves and others - be prepared for denial and possible anger. The bully has a personality characteristic that only they can change. Leave them alone and they will move on to another target.

Do you recognize your own behavior or the behavior of a family member, peer or work colleague in this chapter? Do you feel that this behavior is affecting you or your loved ones?  There are lots of books, web sites and counselors trained to work with bullies and their targets.  Get knowledge and help to change your own behavior whether you are the bully or the target.

Your health is at stake!

# Accepting
# Responsibility is Powerful!

Food for Thought: We are powerless to change behaviors we don't take responsibility for. When we shift blame or make excuses we give away our personal power – the power to make a difference.

It's very important for self growth to be open to suggestion, criticism and change. This is a given. Getting to the point of seeking change requires that we first accept that we and we alone are responsible for our own situation. We are where we are now in our lives because of our past and present behavior.

Psychologists tell us that people who don't take personal responsibility for their behavior run the risk of being:

- Overly dependent on others for recognition, approval, affirmation, and acceptance.

- Chronically hostile, angry, or depressed over how unfairly you have been or are being treated.

- Fearful about ever taking a risk or making a decision.

- Overwhelmed by disabling fears.

- Unsuccessful at the enterprises you take on in life.

- Unsuccessful in personal relationships.

- Emotionally or physically unhealthy.

- Addicted to unhealthy substances, such as the abuse of alcohol, drugs, food, or unhealthy behavior such as excessive gambling, shopping, sex, smoking, work, etc.

- Over responsible and guilt ridden in your need to rescue and enable others in your life.

- Unable to develop trust or to feel secure with others.

- Resistant to vulnerability.

In other words, blaming others or our personal situation for our choices and behaviors leads to all kinds of problems!

Have you heard marriage and relationship counselors say to "Behave like you are in love with your spouse and you will be"? Sounds crazy doesn't it? But, think about the opposite. When someone behaves as if they don't like you, it's pretty easy to associate negative feelings with this person. What do you do? Decide you don't like them? Avoid them? Positive behaviors generate positive feelings. Negative generates negative.

For example:

John and Jane Anyman have been married for 15 years and have a small child. They are both 40 years old and have good careers. Their relationship is good, but having a child adds some conflict. John, however, decides that he isn't happy in his life and begins to behave like he doesn't have a family. He has an affair.

What happens next is predictable. He decides that his marriage was never good and that he is in love with his affair partner. He blames his marriage and Jane for his choices and behaviors. If his happiness means lying, cheating and neglecting his loved ones… he feels entitled to do this. Although Jane doesn't know about the affair, she does feel John's behavior is resentful, angry, selfish and overly critical towards her and their child.

Eventually, John tells Jane about the affair and apologizes. He says that he still wants to be with her BUT doesn't change his behavior. He continues to stay away from home and lie to Jane.

What do you think Jane does? What would you do if you were Jane? Tough question! Jane eventually divorces John. Why? By shifting the blame to "a bad marriage" and "Jane" as the reason for his behavior; John let Jane know that he felt entitled rather than responsible. Worse, John's hurtful BEHAVIOR shows her his true feelings much more than his words.

In modern society, behavior is more important than motive or feelings. For example, does it really matter that the businessman who gives large amounts of money to charity is motivated by publicity rather than just doing a good deed? Is it important that a Nobel Prize is the true motive for the scientist who discovers a vaccine for malaria? The end result is the same. People have been helped. The world is better off. The scientist and businessman feel good about their success and contribution.

Now let's apply this idea to smaller issues. Do you know someone who cannot be depended on to help when needed? Whenever asked, there's a series of boring excuses about why they "can't" do the favor. It's easy to see that they are CHOOSING not to do it for you, isn't it? How does it make you feel? Their behavior, not their words, is showing their true intentions towards you.

As a fitness instructor, I use this idea a lot to get a feel for how serious a client is. Someone who has decided to take responsibility for identifying and changing habits that are deleterious to their health and well-being don't make excessive excuses. They accept that past behavior hasn't worked and are willing to learn new behaviors that will lead to success.

Even though we teach our kids these lessons, true growth and success at any age requires a person to:

Take responsibility for their behavior.

Admit mistakes, without blaming other people or situations.

Change the behavior until they are successful.

This success brings positive feelings, self-esteem, self-respect ... and PERSONAL POWER!

# The Focusing Illusion

A win on the lottery is not the key to enduring happiness, according to researchers in the UK and US who study what makes people happy. Apparently, after the initial euphoria wears off, people return to the same level of happiness they had before the lottery win. There's much speculation among the researchers as to why.

Have you ever heard the term "focusing illusion"? It basically boils down to the idea that when people think about or fantasize about a major life change, we tend to exaggerate the effect the change will have on our happiness. We imagine it will be either far better or far worse than what actually happens after the dust settles from the change. Has this happened to you?

Have you ever worked toward buying something, say a nice car? First you say to yourself, "Boy, I would love to have that car". After a while, you make a decision to save to buy the car. Your thoughts change to "When I have my new car…things will be great!" You save and the day comes to buy the car. It's a wonderful day, you are elated to be behind the wheel of this amazing vehicle and you just know that everyone is envious of you and your flash car. Days and weeks go by. Life continues as usual. It begins to dawn on you that, although you are very happy with the car itself, you are no more happy with life than before you had it.

See how this works?

What about bigger life changes like a new job, new spouse, location change, new baby, etc…?

For those of you who have teens in your home: How often have you heard this? "When I go to university and leave home, things are gonna be much better for me" or similar comments? Well, we parents who went through it already know that while the freedom of growing up is really fun and exciting, there is responsibility associated with it. The initial euphoria of leaving home and being on your own wears off and becomes "normal" or even difficult.

Divorce is another example. If you have been through one (unfortunately, many of us have), you might remember reaching the decision in your mind that you had had "enough". Even if you were not the one who wanted the divorce – you probably got there anyway. With that decision, your mind turns toward the future: how much better your life will be without the other person, how you will be free to find someone better for you, how you will be free of conflict and fighting and, of course, if you are divorcing because you feel you are in love with someone else, how much better your life will be with your new love. And so it goes...

What was the long term reality? My guess? After a few years in your new life, you were the same person as before your problems began. Am I right? Yes, you were unhappy with the SITUATION of your old life; but if you were generally happy within yourself, you remained so. If you were not, once the focusing illusion is gone, you were the same - unhappy.

There is a dark side to the focusing illusion. Do you know someone whose parent, spouse or boss is overly critical? Don't you feel sad or worried for the person? What would you say to them if they asked? Run away – this relationship is not good for you. Yet, this person probably keeps a hold of the focusing illusion "If only I could do this or have this, I would feel loved by my parent, spouse or be rewarded by my boss." This dynamic occurs in many abusive relationships: verbal, emotional and physical. Not healthy. Yet many people propagate this, because of the optimism the focusing illusion provides.

While the focusing illusion can help us work toward a goal, wisdom helps distinguish the reality from the fantasy. Life experiences teach us that external forces (people, situations and material things) cannot "make" us happy or unhappy. Blaming others for our unhappiness or depending on others to provide happiness only serves to alienate everyone close to us. In fact, by believing this we are giving away our personal power of self-determination and our choice to be happy.

The moral of this story?

The focusing illusion serves to motivate people in many ways. It contributes to our ability to dream and remain optimistic in the face of adversity. Dreams drive us forward and give us the power to make our lives magnificent.

To put it in another way: it's not the dreams or desires themselves that make us happy. It's the accomplishments and connections that come with pursuing them with honesty and integrity that is the true root of our happiness.

It's the process of getting there....

# How to Use Criticism as a Learning Tool

One of the qualities I really appreciate my husband Dave for is that he knows how to listen to criticism without defense, evaluate it and use the knowledge. It's easy to see how this life skill (among others) has increased his success in all areas of his life.

Accepting criticism as a chance to improve is a valuable life skill.

In the workplace, we call it feedback. In our personal relationships we call it criticism. Either way, it's the same thing. No matter how it's delivered, the sender is giving us a gift of growth and improvement. It's important, however, to accept feedback without being defensive or blocking it. Not all criticism is valid, but look objectively and you will probably find opportunity buried in the comment.

Everyone loves to learn, but most of us don't like to be taught. Teaching involves criticism. If you are a parent, you have experienced the age old phenomenon of trying to teach your children without criticism so as to bolster their self-esteem. It's harder than it looks, isn't it?

Do you feel like you have trouble accepting criticism? I don't know anyone who likes it, but it's part of the learning experience. Our teachers and mentors do it all the time, and we accept it as part of learning. But what about in our personal lives?

Do you get angry or defensive when someone gives you criticism? Or do you see it as a chance to self-correct and improve? Have you ever given "negative feedback" to someone with good intentions which was met with anger? How did you feel? On the flipside, have you given criticism to someone and be told "You are right. Thank you for telling me"! How did that make you feel?

Have you ever been through counseling? It's tough! Why? Because the counselor leads you through self "evaluation" – to get you to a place where you stop blaming others and see your part in your own unhappiness. If you have done this, I congratulate you. Many people are not brave enough to face self-criticism and follow through with lasting change. After all, it's always easier to blame others for your mistakes. It definitely leads to stagnation.

I looked on the web for suggestions on how to receive criticism and learn from it. I found lots of good information.

Common reasons why we give criticism:

- To help someone improve.

- To see a change that we would like.

- To further the discussion.

- To hurt someone. (destructive)

- To vent our frustrations. (destructive)

- To boost our ego. (destructive)

Some Common Criticism Styles That Hurt:

- Use of insulting or degrading language, or putting down the person.

- Use of focus on the person rather than the action. (eg. "You're a lousy singer")

- Assumption by the listener that what they say or do is always right, and that the criticism is wrong.

How to Use Criticism as a Learning Tool:

- Stop Your First Reaction

- Take a deep breath and think before getting defensive.

- Turn a Negative Into a Positive

- Even with the meanest spirited of criticism you can find honest feedback and a suggestion for improvement.

- Be the Better Person

- Take the criticism of your actions, not your person. Detach emotionally and see if it has validity. Don't attack or defend without pondering.

- Thank the Critic

- Even if someone is harsh and rude, thank them. For you might not have thought about it before!

- Learn from the Criticism. Don't just go back to business as usual. Actually try to do better. Make a change happen.

When you are feeling emotional from someone's criticism, it's helpful to try and remember that most criticism is meant to help. learning to evaluate it objectively will lead to many opportunities for growth and improvement!

# Your Lifestyle
# Changes and Your Family

Jane Doe is turning forty next month. Her husband John and she are healthy and keep regular exercise as part of their lives. They both feel that they eat right and are happy with their bodies. Jane has an office job and teaches fitness classes part-time. John also has a desk job and is a member of a running club.

Jane feels good about herself, but wonders why her fitness routine and healthy diet have not yielded the results she expects. So, in anticipation of being a "forty something", she decides to revamp her exercise and eating to really transform her body. She studies up on new fitness/nutrition science, talks to other fitness instructors and nutritionists, comes up with a plan for herself and implements it.

Although her new plan is not particularly difficult, it does require that she be more disciplined in her eating habits, eating schedules and the way she works out. After her research, she realizes that truly attaining the body transformation that she wants requires more than just doing what she has done year after year. In fact, it's yielding diminishing returns!

When Jane first explains to John what she intends to do, John is very support-ive. He thinks it's important for Jane to feel good about herself especially at this time in her life. Deep down, however, John feels that Jane will "mellow out" and return to her previous behavior soon enough. So, any inconvenience to him caused by her lifestyle change is temporary…right?

Fast forward a few months. Jane has worked out her dietary needs, schedules and foods quite nicely. Her workouts are coming along and she is starting to see real change. She likes it…

John, on the other hand, has always felt that he is the fitter one. After all, his friends always ask his advice about workouts and fitness. His routine hasn't changed in 10 years, though, and he really doesn't think about the quality of the food he eats. His attitude is that so long as he exercises, he can eat what he wants. He has accepted his slowly growing "love handles" as part of aging. But now, he seems to be getting older and Jane seems to be getting younger!

Fast forward six more months....Jane is really looking and feeling different. She has remained true to her goals and everyone comments to her how amazing the changes are. After all, she was already "fit" before. When she and John go out, John can see how men are attracted to her like they were when she was 15 years younger. She exudes a confidence that he hasn't seen in years.

John is starting to feel insecure with his own body, his own fitness accomplishments and even his attractiveness to Jane! He wishes that she would go back to being the wonderful, "soft" woman she used to be instead of the hard-body babe she is becoming. He begins to feel resentment and jealousy of her attention and success.

John has two choices here. He can learn from Jane's experience, try some things for himself and transform his body; or he can continue to believe that Jane's methods are too extreme and resent her success.

If you are over age 35, you probably know more than one couple with a similar story as Jane and John. You might even have had the same experience yourself. A physical transformation by one partner in a couple and not the other can lead to adjustment problems.

The message is that we as individuals are solely responsible for our own physical fitness and health. However, changes in eating behaviors, work out schedules and interests do affect the people closest to us in a variety of ways. Sometimes, like John, resentment develops in the unchanging partner. Sometimes competition fuels this, sometimes fear, sometimes a feeling of inadequacy, or not understanding how important it is to the other partner.

So, if you are the transformer, it's important to listen to your partner and empathize with the difficulties your lifestyle and physical changes are causing. As you transform, be aware of the insecurities that might arise because you are moving in a new direction and reassure your partner whenever you have the chance.

If you are the partner who is not currently in the process of body transformation, talk about the inconveniences, feelings and insecurities you have. Ask your partner why he/she feels the need to change so dramatically. Communicate your feelings!

# Get Smart!

As I was doing some research for this chapter the other day, I came across a rather disturbing idea....that the brain starts it's age related decline after age 30! After doing some quick mental math (let's see, um, I am 47 years old now, minus 30..) I realized that my brain has been declining for 17 years! Bummer.

There is an encouraging side to this news. New research indicates that exercise makes older people smarter by slowing age-related brain decline.

Many of you have probably heard about the study reported in the journal Nature in 1999 which studied previously sedentary people over the age of 60. Those who walked vigorously for 45 minutes three days a week significantly improved their mental processing abilities that usually decline with age. I remember reading about this study back in '99 and thinking that it makes sense. After all, I know quite a few active older people who are "still sharp as a tack", as my Mom would say.

In 2003, a new study was released which added fuel to this idea that exercise helps keep brain aging at bay. This study was sponsored by the National Institute on Aging, part of the United States National Institute of Health. In this study, researchers studied well educated adults aged 55 to 79 by taking brain scans (MRI) of participants and by putting this together with findings from previous research. The results were very enlightening.

The MRI scans showed significant differences in the brains of the fitter individuals. What's more, both the learning and memory stuff (grey matter) and the signal transmission bits (white matter) were denser in the fitter folks. Although the researchers used the words "improved cognitive function" to describe the results of the findings, what these findings say to me is that the fitter participants learn faster, think faster and remember better. Pretty cool stuff.

Another interesting thing about this study is the comparison of brain density of older fit people.

That is to say that fitness in and of itself does not seem to be a predictor of brain density. When taken in the context of fit people over 30, however, the brain differences were significant.

Some other interesting things that the researchers noticed were that participants who exercised more than 30 minutes per day had the most benefit. The most effective "brain-building" exercise method used by participants was a combination of aerobics and weight training. Women on hormone replacement therapy showed more brain benefit from exercise than those not on the therapy.

So...the next time you don't feel like working out, just remember that moving your body makes your brain work better too. Now that's time well spent don't you think?

Look good and get smart!

# HEALTH

# Health Habit Sabotage

So, you've been working out regularly and are really starting to see changes in your body. But, for some reason you feel tired, without energy and are getting more colds than usual. Your doctor says you are in good health. So, what's up with this tired feeling? It's time to look at the other aspects of wellness involved. In other words, are your lifestyle choices and habits sabotaging your good work at the gym?

Let's take a look at a few things that can affect your health and wellbeing and hence your fitness:

1. **Procrastination**

   Procrastination can really wreak havoc on your health. For example, if you put off your exercise day after day, you lose fitness. If you put off going to the doctor for an illness, it's likely to get worse. But what about everyday tasks? If you put them off, they end up having to be completed in a hurry, you end up stressed and have to put off other things (like sleep and exercise) for a few days.

2. **Losing weight by eating less often**

   I have to admit, I am guilty of this one from time to time. It never works. Basically, your body needs the fuel on a regular basis or it goes into starvation mode, saves calories and doesn't burn them. This not only makes you feel tired, but it also lowers your immune system.

3. **Taking too much on/ chronic stress**

   Stress is an individual thing. I have friends who have full-time jobs, go to school part-time and have small children. For me, this is overwhelming and I know a lifestyle like that would make me seriously stressed out. But one thing for sure about stress on a long term basis... it impacts the body in many ways, not the least of which is the immune system.

4. **Not sleeping enough/catching up on weekends**
It's really important to get enough sleep with REGULARITY (the experts call this good sleep hygiene). The body and brain requires adequate sleep to rebuild and regenerate. Without solid rest, the body just doesn't recover from that really hard work- out, or really stressful business trip and you end up feeling a bit weaker or even catching a cold.

5. **Working out too much/not recovering**
This is really important if you are training for a sports event or want to improve your muscle development in the gym. Muscles need rest in between workouts (see sleep above as well) to rebuild from whatever loads you put on them. If they become too fatigued, the joints end up taking the stress of the activity... which can end in injury and weakness. Your immune system is also compromised by long or hard workouts and needs time to recover.

6. **Holding on to anger**
The way people process anger has a big impact on their body. The classic example of this is the "Type A" personality type who has a heart attack. I am not really qualified to discuss this in depth, but anger has an evolutionary reason (flight or fight response) which is necessary. But the body responses to anger are designed to be short in duration. Holding on to anger keeps the body in this state. Eventually, health is compromised.

Wishing you good health and fitness always!

# What Can You Do to Reduce Your Cancer Risk?

The more research that is done on the different types of cancers, the more it becomes evident that there's a lot of risk that can be controlled by lifestyle changes. Most of us already know that smoking causes cancer, but there are some other lifestyle factors that may or may not be so obvious.

### Smoking

Don't smoke. Don't hang out with people who do smoke.

Study after study shows that secondhand smoke is equally as damaging to health as is you smoked yourself. It's not just the smoke.

Basically, cigarette smoke contains 69 known cancer causing chemicals and hundreds of other poisons. Some of these lovely chemicals include arsenic, benzene, cadmium, formaldehyde, polonium and cyanide. Sounds great huh?

Since we are talking about cancer prevention, I don't think I need to mention the significant increase in heart disease and stroke of smokers or that smoker's tend to look older because the skin is deprived of adequate oxygen.

### Chemical Exposure

The average person is exposed to 126 chemicals per day in their personal care products alone!

In addition, we are exposed to chemicals in our work environment, home environment, pesticides and environmental pollutants in our food.

Scientists point not so much to any single chemical but the cocktail of chemicals that we are exposed to on a regular basis as contributors.

### Food

A diet high in smoked meats, fish, cured or pickled foods increases risk for cancer. Too many fried and fatty foods is also a bad idea (see body weight below).

The US Department of Agriculture recommends eating a wide variety of foods to avoid overexposure to pesticides, fertilizers used to produce the food or environmental pollutants present in the food.

### Alcohol

Men who consume more than 2 drinks per day and women who drink more than 1 raise their cancer risk significantly.

Heavy alcohol use messes with the body's hormones.

### Sun safety

Skin cancer is still on the rise. Wearing sun screen and avoiding prolonged exposure especially in the middle of the day lowers your risk.

It also has the added benefit of keeping your skin younger and healthier looking much later in life!

### Body weight

An overweight body is at increased risk not only for cancers but heart disease, diabetes and a host of other problems.

Extra body fat can lead to an excess of certain hormones and hence increased risk for hormone dependent cancers.

### Exercise

Being active helps keep the body's hormones in balance and body fat in check. See above.

### Sex

Exposure to the HPV virus through an infected partner can lead to cancer. Condoms are a help but do not prevent transmission of this virus.

Exposure to Hepatitis C can lead to liver cancer as well.

### Family Health History

Some cancers do have a genetic component such as colon and breast cancer.

It's important to have regular checks if you have a family member who develops cancer.

### Regular Cancer Screening

Get the recommended checkups regularly. Early detection is key as many cancers are curable if caught early enough.

Pretty simple stuff. Small changes, big rewards!

# Taking Charge of
# Your Own Healthcare

I am American by birth, culture and nationality, but I haven't lived there for 19 years. In 1988, chasing adventure and work, I left the states. Since then, I have lived all over the world moving every few years. Currently, I live in Singapore.

As an "expat"(person who chooses to live outside their home country), life has its challenges. One of which is that one has to be very diligent in taking charge of the healthcare needs of oneself and family.

All in all, I have had very good luck with the docs I have seen over the years. Of course, except for having a baby, I haven't developed any medical conditions requiring care – just the odd flu or injury etc. It has been my experience that physicians the world over are a learned and caring group. The problems seem to arise because of communication (or lack there of). Many doctors have been taught to diagnose and treat, but not explain to the patient the details of their condition. So it's up to the patient to be informed enough to ask.

Every place has its own healthcare system, with unique organizational structures and standards of care…some extremely good and easy, like Singapore, and some not so good or easy. My last assignment was a small town in Borneo (yes, the place that used to have head hunters!). There were good doctors there but it was up to me to find those that I could work and communicate with.

Over the years, I developed a system where I would go to a doctor, get a diagnosis, read about it in the Merck Manual, research the web (more recent years), then go back to the doctor and ask more questions. The system resulted not only in the expansion of my knowledge about me and my family's health, but also development of close connections to my physicians. I am sure most of them thought of me as either an overly enthusiastic patient or generally an annoyance – but I got attention!

A while back I was reading an article by Barbara Morris, the author of "Put Old on Hold", where she talks about how Americans in what she calls second middle age (60, 70's and beyond) need to take an active role in their own healthcare and prevention. So, it's not just an issue for someone who moves around a lot....

It's important for each of us to be fully informed of any medical conditions that we might have, what the side effects of medications that we are prescribed might be, what allergies we have and the genetic predispositions that we might have (like a parent with diabetes or certain cancers). It's also crucial to be very candid with a new doctor about one's medical history and such.

Since I left the states 19 years ago, the American medical system has changed to "managed care". This is a system that I am not familiar with, but it looks like it requires much more patient involvement than the medical system of 20 years ago. Also, I would speculate that doctors have learned to be much more specific in explaining to patients about their care and medical conditions because of this. In my opinion, this is a good thing because as patients know more they can make informed decisions and action on prevention and treatment.

I wonder, though, has the "managed care" way of doing things resulted in patient cost savings – its original intent?

I recently renewed my medical insurance policy. I was given 2 pricing options for the SAME coverage. One was for people who spend the majority of their time in the U.S. or live there and the other was for people who live and spend most of their time anywhere else in the world. No kidding – the U.S. coverage was 4 times as expensive as the non-US. 4 times!!

Wow...no wonder healthcare costs in the US make international news.

I will get off the soapbox now and let someone else talk. Take care of yourself and your loved ones!

# Lifestyles, Behaviors and Lower Risk of Death

According to the Center for Disease Control in the United States, the life expectancy for American men is 75 (74.5) and women is 80 (79.9). The top killers for men and top killers for women are pretty similar.   Here's the list.  You may be surprised:

For American Men, the top 8 causes of death over a lifetime are:

      No. 1 — Heart disease
      No. 2 — Cancer
      No. 3 — Accidents (unintentional injuries)
      No. 4 — Stroke
      No. 5 — Chronic obstructive pulmonary disease (COPD)
      No. 6 — Diabetes
      No. 7 — Pneumonia and influenza
      No. 8 — Suicide

For American Women, the top 8 causes of death over a lifetime are:

      No. 1 — Heart disease
      No. 2 — Cancer
      No. 3 — Stroke
      No. 4 — Chronic obstructive pulmonary disease (COPD)
      No. 5 — Alzheimer's disease
      No. 6 — Diabetes
      No. 7 — Accidents
      No. 8 — Pneumonia and influenza

It's important to note that these "killers" are over a lifetime, and that the major causes of death shift within certain age groups.

If you are a woman in your 20s, accidents are your biggest risk factor for death. Likewise, from ages 35 to 64, your greatest risk is cancer. For men, from childhood until age 44, accidents are the most significant threat. From 55 to 64, cancer is the biggest cause of death.

Lung cancer is still by far the biggest cancer killer in both sexes. 90% of this cancer is caused by cigarettes. Prostate, colorectal and breast cancer, the other leading cancers have all been associated with high fat diets, overweight and lack of exercise. Smoking is also a primary contributor for chronic obstructive pulmonary disease (COPD).

More than twice as many men as women die each year in traffic accidents. Male drivers involved in such accidents are almost twice as likely as female drivers to be intoxicated.

Surprisingly, men commit suicide four times as often as women do. Depression is estimated to affect 7 percent of men in any given year and is a risk factor for suicide. Substance abuse, more common in men, can mask depression.

More women than men have Alzheimer's. In fact, women die of it at more than twice the rate that men do. One reason may be that women generally live longer, and the risk of Alzheimer's increases with age.

Putting all this together, the lifestyle behaviors you can employ to lessen your chances of dying of the big killers or at least putting them off look like this:

1. Avoid smoking, using other tobacco products and exposure to passive smoke.
2. Limit the amount of alcohol you drink.
3. Eat a diet rich in fruits, vegetables and whole-grain products.
4. Exercise regularly.
5. Control other health conditions that may put a strain on your heart, such as high blood pressure, diabetes and high cholesterol.
6. Maintain a healthy weight.
7. Limit saturated fats.
8. Be aware of potential cancer-causing substances (carcinogens) in your home and workplace, and take steps to reduce your exposure to these substances.
9. Have regular preventive health screenings.
10. Know your family medical history and review it with your doctor.
11. Use your seat belt.
12. Keep your speed down when driving.
13. Don't drive while sleepy or under the influence of drugs or alcohol.
14. Limit your exposure to sun and use sunscreen.

Nothing really new or earth shattering, just common sense!

# Is it Perfume or Poison?

Here's the scenario: you are on an elevator. The elevator stops and in walks someone with WAY too much cologne on and the smell overpowers you. Your sinuses start to hurt and you get a bit sick to your stomach. The smell of the cologne stays with you, in your hair, clothes and nose for quite a while after — hence the sick feeling does too.

Yuk. It's hard not to think how inconsiderate this person is.

It's not just the smell that is inconsiderate. Have you ever thought about the chemicals that are used in fragrances? Many of them are not good for you to breathe or to put on your body!

This week Time Magazine did an article on air fresheners and how many brands have been removed from the market due to high levels of phthalates? Phthalates are estrogenic in nature, which is believed to contribute to certain cancers. Phthalates are used to dissolve and carry fragrances and soften plastics, sealants and similar compounds. They are commonly found in cosmetics, paint, nail polish and plastics.

This peaked my interest on fragrances in general — so, as usual, I did some research.

Although fragrances have been used for centuries, they were made from plant and animal sources. Modern fragrances are primarily synthetic materials developed since World War II.

Did you know that 600 or more chemicals may be used in a single fragrance, and 95% of chemicals used in them are derived from petroleum? Why? Petro-chemicals in perfumes are less expensive and more easily available than the natural ingredients.

Many chemicals used in fragrances are considered hazardous waste disposal chemicals! Synthetic fragrance compounds accumulate in human tissue and are found in breast milk.

An EPA study in 1991 listed the 20 most common chemicals used in "fragrance products" which are used not only in perfumes but to scent shampoos, soaps, deodorants, lotions, creams and other beauty products. Here's the list – it speaks volumes on its own:

1. Acetone
2. Benzaldehyde
3. Benzyl
4. Benzyl Alcohol
5. Camphor
6. Ethanol
7. Ethyl Acetate
8. Limonene
9. Linalool
10. Methylene Chloride
11. a-Pinene
12. g-Terpinene
13. a-Terpineol
14. 1,8-Cineole
15. b-Citronellol
16. b-Myrcene
17. Nerol
18. Ocimene
19. b-Phenethyl Alcohol
20. a-Terpinolene

There are relatively few studies available concerning the use and exposure to fragranced products. Testing by the cosmetics/fragrance industry focuses on skin effects without taking into account respiratory, neurological, or systemic effects. There is little regulation of fragrance by regulatory agencies.

Not only is too much perfume often offensive to many, more and more people consider it to be an indoor air pollutant. Some are quite vocal about their opposition to the use of perfumes. For years, I thought I was the only one who got headaches from strong perfume!

There is a movement afoot to curtail the use of fragrances in the work place. Many businesses, at the request of their employees, are creating fragrance-free policies. Given that many people are highly affected by allergies, this makes sense (pun intended, get it? ... sense...scents...).

But seriously, given that we are bombarded by more and more hazardous chemicals and pollution, having less on our bodies, homes and in our workplaces must be better for ALL of us.

Breathe deeply and live well!

# Take Care of Your Heart

The American Heart Association strives to educate people about how to stay well and keep their hearts in shape. They challenge people to address general wellness factors and give them ideas on how to do it. In general, they urge awareness of how to recognize heart problems and strokes, what to do if you have symptoms, how to assess personal risk factors, get regular medical check ups, regular exercise, healthy eating habits and not smoking.

Ok. We all know we should exercise, eat "right", have regular medical checks and lower stress levels. Let's look at some of the current dietary and exercise recommendations specifically aimed at maintaining a healthy heart. After all, the more research the medical folks do, the more they change what the "right" things to do are!

Exercise is pretty simple: at least 30 minutes of moderately rigorous exercise most or all days of the week.

Interestingly, the type of exercise makes little difference in terms of heart health. Weight training has proven to be heart healthy as well as more aerobic activities. No matter what you enjoy, just stay moving!!!

Nutrition is not so simple. Some of the newer recommendations include:

- Eat LOTS of vegetables, some fruit, whole grains and lean protein.

- Add Omega-3 fats, which come from fish oil, nuts, seeds and some oils.

- Eat much less processed foods because they contain trans fats which are more harmful to the heart than saturated fats!

- Fry food much less often. Frying food changes the structure of fat molecules (trans fats) and degrades protein.

- The heart needs B-vitamins to keep it healthy. Processed grains (white flour, rice, etc) lose 60-90% of the vitamins in processing. Eat brown and unprocessed where possible.

- Keep desserts and sweets to a minimum.

- Add a multivitamin, just to make sure to get necessary nutrients (especially B vitamins).

Wellness Issues:

- Learn to cope with stress, communicate better, manage anger etc. Repressed emotions are terrible for the heart as well as overall health (and cause relationship problems too).

- Stop smoking.

- Control alcohol intake.

- Be aware of direct relatives who have had heart disease or Type 2 diabetes (a risk factor for heart attacks)

- If you have Type 2 diabetes, follow your physician's instructions!

- Keep your body fat at normal levels.

So, this Valentine's Day, when you are feeling your most romantic....show your partner how much you love him/her by making resolutions to become more heart healthy by the time the next Valentine's Day comes around. Taking care of your body so you will be around for your partner a long time is soooo romantic ..... and sexy!

# Green Cleaning Ideas for Your Home

When my husband, Dave, and I first started housekeeping together, he used to shake his head and occasionally comment on my refusal to use artificial chemical cleaning products in the home. Yes, it is a bit unconventional to say the least! But even he will tell you that he likes that our house is free of toxic chemicals.

Only ten years ago, I too believed the only way to really clean was with smelly household cleaners. Here's the story:

Have you heard of the hygiene hypothesis? First proposed in England in 1989 by David Strachan, it was a possible explanation of why kids raised in larger families have a lower incidence of allergies. It has been studied extensively and has now been expanded.

The current thinking is that early exposure to bacteria, viruses, parasites etc. are important for the development of a healthy immune system. This is a radical shift in thinking from the antibacterial paradigm most of us were raised with years ago.

Ten years ago, I had a baby. I was living in England at the time. The medical community there was beginning to discuss and apply this new hygiene paradigm. I was encouraged to breast feed, of course, but also to not worry so much about sterilizing bottles and utensils after the baby was a few months old.

Naturally, as an over tired new parent, when the hygiene hypothesis was explained to me, I happily followed along. It did make a lot of sense. After all, babies have lived for thousands of years with lots and lots of dirt around and have thrived. Besides, sterilizing everything WAS a lot of work....

Well, guess what? At age 10, that same child rarely gets sick and has no allergies so far...even with a genetic predisposition to asthma from both parents!

For me the hygiene hypothesis paradigm shift led to a "re-think" about all the chemicals and insecticides that were being used in and around the house to keep it clean and "pest" free. It's really quite incredible what a young child and parents are exposed to in terms of household chemicals these days. The question is why? If early exposure to microbes is good for baby – why expose a child to pollutants in the name of killing them?

So, the search for healthier alternatives began....

Through trial and error and speaking with other parents who have gone in favor of "green cleaning", I learned that pretty much all household cleaning can be done using a bit of creativity and things you already have in your kitchen. Using greener alternatives is easy, inexpensive, good for your family and good for the earth.

Here are some ideas:

- **Baking soda:** Acts as a scrub, polishes metal and deodorizes things. (a must have if you have a baby in diapers).

- **Lemon:** Deodorizes, cuts grease, bleaches stains and disinfects. Mixed with baking soda, it removes stains from plastic food storage containers.

- **Salt:** Another scrubber (more course than baking soda)—good for cookware and ovens. Combined with citrus juice it removes rust.

- **White vinegar:** Deodorizes and disinfects (again acid). Mix with water and a little dish soap and you've got a great all purpose cleaner for windows, floors, bathrooms and all the rest. Used full strength it fights mold and mildew and body odor in clothing.

- **Olive Oil:** Mix two parts oil with one part lemon juice and use as a furniture polish. It smells great.

So, if you are thinking of going organic with the food you eat, why not go all the way and get rid of the pollutants in your house. You and your family will benefit with better health and more pocket money. If you have children – you won't have to worry about poisoning. After all, what's the worst thing that can happen from drinking vinegar except a tummy ache?

And, when you say you can eat off the floor in your home, you will really mean it!

# Is Bottled Water Really Better?

Do you drink bottled water because you believe to be a healthier option than your local tap water? You might want to re-think this. Tests on leading brands of bottled water turned up a variety of contaminants often found in tap water, according to a recently published 2-year long study by the Environmental Working Group in the U.S.

The bottled water did not turn out to be much better than tap water -and in some cases worse.

The study's lab tests on 10 brands of bottled water detected 38 chemicals including bacteria, caffeine, the pain reliever acetaminophen, fertilizer, solvents, plastic-making chemicals and the radioactive element strontium. Though some probably came from tap water that some companies use for their bottled water, other contaminants probably leached from plastic bottles, the researchers said.

"In some cases, it appears bottled water is no less polluted than tap water and, at 1,900 times the cost, consumers should expect better," said Jane Houlihan, an environmental engineer who co-authored the study.

Ok. Let's explore this further. The bottlers take already polluted tap water, "purify" it with a carbon filter, reverse osmosis or even distillation (the purest). Then the water is put back into disposable plastic bottles where it may remain in the plastic on the store shelves for weeks. Chemicals from the plastic leach back into the water and can create an even more hazardous potion. Not to mention any bacteria that may come off the equipment or the hands of the people working in the plant multiply over time in the bottles.

What a bargain!

Hmm... and this is in the US! What about other parts of the world where industrial pollution is not regulated like the US? My family and I live in Malaysia. The water is chlorinated here, so there's not much risk of bacterial infection - but the chemicals in the ground water from poorly regulated and unreported industrial activities is cause for worry.

An example of this is a pesticide free vegetable farm in nearby Singapore that we visited a year ago. During the tour, the guide stated that, for ethical reasons, the farm did not actually call itself organic because they didn't know what the land in the area had been used for 15 years before. Hence, they didn't have a complete picture of what pollutants are in the soil. Yet, the farm next door had a big sign stating it was "organic"!

Convenience can be a good reason to buy bottled water; but why not consider purifying your own? At least then, you know where it came from! You can store the water in glass which is less likely to leach pollutants back into the water. It's simple to do and much less expensive. There are tons of brands of purifiers and filters for you to choose from.

At our house, we distill our water and use a Brita brand carbon filter. The distilled water is very pure (which makes a wonderful tasting coffee) but requires a fair bit of electricity. The Brita filter removes only some of the chemicals and pollutants but is only a matter of pouring the tap water into the jug through a filter. Simple, fast and inexpensive. In many places, you can also purchase 5 gallon glass bottles of water purified in your preferred way for home delivery which is convenient and a bit more cost effective than the individual plastic bottles.

Stay hydrated!

# Sugar Feeds Cancer?

Is there a link between sugar consumption and cancer? Seventy years ago, Otto Warburg won a Nobel Prize for his discovery of glucose as the fuel that grows cancer cells. In other words, sugar feeds cancer. Ok, this makes sense. All of our body's tissues use glucose for fuel.

First, some boring stuff. A few new studies have followed along these lines and have associated sugar consumption with several types of cancer: A study done on women in Mexico linked high carbohydrate diets with breast cancer. The same link was made by a study done on American women.

A small study at University of Southern California identified a significant increase in risk for small bowel cancer in people who consumed the most sugar in coffee, tea and non-diet sodas. (Not the purpose of the study. It was chance finding).

A Harvard School of Public Health study demonstrated that a diet high in simple carbohydrate foods such as white rice, white bread and white potatoes increased risk of pancreatic cancer in overweight and sedentary women. Besides cigarette smoking, this is the first risk factor identified with pancreatic cancer. Colorectal cancer risk has been linked to higher insulin levels, as well.

This pancreatic cancer study findings make sense. The pancreas produces insulin – the hormone that helps the body utilize blood glucose. Overweight people tend to be "insulin resistant". This means the pancreas works harder producing more insulin. It's a vicious cycle.

Here's some food for thought. Cancer rates have increased over the last 100 years or so. Mostly, this is attributed to increased cigarette smoking (there's no arguing that this is the single most risk factor for many types of cancers, not only lung), and arguably the presence of more industrial chemicals and pollution.

Let's look at the consumption of sugar over the same period. In 1815, the average per capita consumption of sugar in Great Britain was 15 pounds per year.

By 1974, the consumption had risen to 120 pounds per year. Holy cow – that's a lot of desserts!

Nowadays, in the US, the average per person yearly amount is 150 pounds per year. This is NOT including corn syrup and high fructose corn syrup which is the stuff that sweetens soft drinks. The average American drinks 34 gallons of soft drinks per year. Ugly statistics.

It's also worthy to note that the use of refined white flour started in the early 1800's in Europe. The rice that is so popular in Southeast Asian cuisine (highly processed) because of its color and quick cooking properties started to be widely used after World War 2. Is there an increase in cancers due to these dietary changes? It would logically follow. Both white rice and white flour cause a blood sugar spike similar to white sugar. Diets high in white rice and white flour, known as refined carbohydrates are associated with increased incidence of Type II Diabetes. Not to mention the nutritional value is very poor because of processing. It is known that the fiber that is in brown rice and brown flour has protective effect against certain cancers including pancreatic and...Type II diabetes. Hmmm.

More and more, nutritionally oriented doctors are saying to cancer patients that cutting down on sugar and refined carbohydrates could slow the growth of the cancer (given that "sugar fuels cancer"). But the real science is not concrete enough for the medical community to say unequivocally that carbs increase cancer cell multiplication.

Since sugar gives you no nutrition (vitamins, minerals, etc) makes the body fat and causes cavities, it can't be good. Doctors, nutritionists and scientists may be divided on the subject, but you can bet that I will be eating "brown" and looking out for hidden sugar in food as much as possible. It looks like "the writing is on the wall"....

# Slim People at Risk for
# Fat Related Health Problems?

Do you assume that because someone is thin that they are also fit? Well, hold on to your hat, researchers are saying that many thin people have the same heart disease risk and type 2 diabetes risk as obese people. In fact, they say that some thin people are at higher risk than sumo wrestlers! The reason? Intra-abdominal fat.

According to Dr. Jimmy Bell, a professor of molecular imaging at Imperial College London, "being thin doesn't automatically mean you're not fat". It's what's inside that makes a difference to your health. Internal fat surrounding vital organs such as the heart and liver can be as dangerous as the fat that you see. Since 1994, Dr. Bell and his colleagues have been mapping the fat stores of people to show where people store fat. They have scanned and recorded more than 800 people.

When most people gain weight, the fat is subcutaneous and we see it. We have known for years that a person who gains fat around the middle of their body is at increased risk for heart disease etc., but this was viewed as an obesity related issue. Now, it's clear that even thin people are at risk. Of the women scanned in the study, 45% of those with normal body mass indices (BMI) had excessive levels of internal fat. Of the men? 60%!

Dr. Bell's research indicates that people who control their weight with diet rather than exercise are likely to have major deposits of fat around their internal organs, no matter how slim they appear on the outside. This leads us to the idea that exercise is the key to controlling levels of fat you can see and fat you can't see.

What's the difference in the health risks of subcutaneous fat and intra-abdominal fat? The metabolic characteristics of intra-abdominal fat are different from subcutaneous fat (the stuff you see). Intra-abdominal fat releases free fatty acids to drain directly into the liver, whereas subcutaneous fat drains into the systemic circulation. The influx of free fatty acids in the liver results in overproduction of very low density lipoprotein, and retention of low density lipoprotein, the "bad cholesterols" in the bloodstream. This can also lead to a lower level of high density lipoprotein, the "good cholesterol".

This research offers a possible explanation for, while the population in developing South East Asian countries still have lower rates of obesity, have a high per capita incidence of Type II diabetes and heart disease. Of course, smoking is still prevalent in this region as well...

What to do? Exercise and eat healthily! And remember... Muscles burn fat. Around age 35, unless maintained through exercise, the body begins to lose muscle and gain fat. Since muscles require energy where as fat cells act as energy storage, a person who stays slim by dieting will require fewer calories as they lose muscle. Over the years, the metabolism slows down because the body has less muscle to burn energy. Any extra energy will be stored as fat somewhere even if it's not visible to the naked eye. If the muscle mass is maintained, the body will simply use fat rather than store it.

It's a simple concept, really.... Dieting may keep a body slim; but healthy eating and a combination of aerobic and resistance exercise keeps a body slim, strong and disease resistant. Hmmm...just more proof that exercise keeps you younger.

# LIFE

# Dating Again After 20 Years –
# An Internet Fairytale

Just imagine for a moment that you and your spouse have split up after a very long marriage. You did not envision this change. You are shocked with the intensity and weight of your own emotions – a painful combination of grief, anger, fear, humiliation, disbelief, sadness, failure, disappointment and others.

You spend hundreds of hours, reading about how to win your spouse back, getting counseling to help with your grief, journaling, making lists of what you did wrong and trying to talk with your spouse about "fixing" things.

Meanwhile, your spouse treats you like someone with a highly contagious fatal disease and looks at you as if you smell like cow manure.

Little by little you wake up to the fact that your life has changed. It's a done deal. There's no going back. You begin to see that by resisting change, you haven't noticed the opportunities opening up before you.

This awakening flows over you like warm sunshine. The heavy feelings of fear and loss are replaced by the lightness of freedom and optimism. Suddenly, the future looks brighter and the present feels sweet.

With new perspective, you change your behavior.

You focus on those things in your life that are special to you – your children, family, friends, job, hobbies and interests long forgotten. You read about finding new love and making successful relationships.

Your lists and journal entries change to what you did not receive from your previous relationship, what you want from your next relationship, what qualities you want in your next partner, what you have to offer a new partner, etc…

You begin to take an interest in YOU. You are excited about the process of creating your future. The past no longer holds you hostage. The past is no longer who you are or who you want to be.

After some time, you feel ready for the D-word...Dating!

Dating...uh, how to begin? It's been a long time since your last date. Oh boy, you are nervous! You read about it, talk to friends about it and start hanging out with single people. Maybe you go clubbing more or join a singles activity.

From dating and relationship reading, you already know that seeking lasting love is a numbers game. It takes time. The early dating experiences allow you to "get your feet wet" - help you learn about what you do and don't want.

You already made up your mind: no compromise in building the relationship you want just to avoid being alone. You will not "settle" for the first available and willing person that comes along. No way!

Then, you find someone you are attracted to and you two decide to "have lunch".

The day of your first date arrives. The excitement makes your stomach feel full of butterflies. At the restaurant, your date is waiting. Things go smoothly until this person mentions that they are married with 2 young children. Strike 3 – the batter is out! You kindly explain that obviously you both are not looking for the same kind of relationship and that you apologize for any misunderstanding. Yuk. Bad start.

The second date goes better. Your date is really hot, but there is one teeny-weeny, microscopic problem. You two don't speak the same language. "Never mind", you say to yourself, "I speak a little of the other person's language and they speak some of mine. And, we have the same profession". Alas, it plays out like this:

Date 1 goes very well. You are on top of the world.

Date 2 goes well, but, you are starting to run out of things to talk about.

Date 3 just gets quiet and uncomfortable.

Your date may be hot, but your conversations run cold.

These sorts of dating experiences continue. You are happy in the new life you have made for yourself and don't feel lonely. You enjoy your dates, have fun and spend time with friends.

One day, you put your profile and picture on an internet dating site. Oh, what fun it turns out to be!

You begin connecting with people all over the world and making even more friends. You are surprised at the quality people that you meet along the way. After all, you had heard how only desperate people use the internet for dating.

Soon, you are meeting internet acquaintances for coffee or dinner. You feel fantastic about the whole thing. Over and over you meet high quality, successful and confident people using the internet dating site. You feel that, for you, the internet is a much better place to meet potentials than by going out clubbing.

Time goes by. You meet many wonderful people, have great times and grow as a person. You think "Hmm. it's not bad at all being single. In fact, I like it a lot!"

Then, you see a profile on the dating web site you haven't seen before. It really stands out as the profile of someone special. The words are magnetic to you. You contact this person and they reply.

The two of you bounce emails back and forth for a couple of weeks and then you start phoning each other. The more the two of you learn about each other, the more connected you feel. You feel that this person is looking for the same things in a romance that you are; and has the emotional maturity, loyalty and integrity required to make a romantic partnership work long-term.

It dawns on you that this person has many of the qualities on your list that you are looking for in a potential partner.

Over time, your phone friendship evolves into a romance...complete with physical chemistry. How can this be? You haven't even been in the same room with this person....

The day arrives and you meet for the first time. The person looks better than their picture, better than you expected...and the attraction feels like burning jet fuel. The relationship has a fiery yet smooth take off and climbs higher and higher and......

Is there a moral to this story? Absolutely!

- Change happens whether you like it or not.

- The quicker you stop resisting change, the quicker you start enjoying it.

- There are tons of opportunities for love out there, even if you are 40, 50, 60 and beyond.

- Don't settle for less than fantastic, just to avoid being alone.

- Look around to find quality people...even in unconventional places.

- Be open and ready to accept love when it hits you over the head!

I learned this firsthand. It was my happy BEGINNING.

# Pets and Stress

My mother used to say "you can always trust a person who has animal hair on them". As a kid, I often pondered what this statement means. Are people who care for animals more trustworthy? Kinder? Gentler?

Well, a recent scientific study says that people who own pets are less stressed. Maybe not more trustworthy, but less stress WOULD indicate greater wellness. An idea worth considering.

The study examined the cardiovascular reactivity when exposed to psychological stress of 240 married couples, half of whom owned a pet. The researchers exposed the people to stressful situations (mental arithmetic problems and stuff like that) in a variety of social support conditions: alone, with pet or friend (friend present for non-pet owners), with spouse, with spouse and pet/friend. They found that the people with the pets had much lower rise in heart rate under such conditions; better than with their spouse or friends.

This evidence the healing help pets provide has been anecdotal for years. Hospitals, retirement homes and other caring facilities have used pets to help promote wellness with a lot of success. So it's no surprise, especially where children are involved.

Over the last couple of weeks, I have conducted my own experiment by observing how the people in my family and visitors to my home relate to my cat and, of course how my cat relates to them.

My cat is a rather funny looking, very playful and affectionate youngish cat named Tony. He is a "hairless" breed, called Sphinx.

Tony has many jobs. One is to help me to write by sitting on my lap and purring loudly. He also reminds me to take breaks by standing up and walking on the computer keyboard! I digress.

One observation that is true for all unknowing participants in my "experiment": everyone that enters my house, friends, family members and even the

FedEx guy, upon seeing Tony, their face changes and becomes somehow softer. It's as if just seeing the cat makes them less stressed. Even the little girl who is very frightened of cats loves to watch the cat from a distance.

My husband, a high energy executive of a multi-national company, is of particular interest to this study. When he arrives home after work or travel, his body language is "Mr. corporate leader". After greeting and kissing his people family members, he looks a bit more relaxed. But it's after he picks up Tony and strokes him (usually followed by giving him some cat food), that he appears to really relax and turn off from work.

Last week, I had a friend over who says she doesn't like cats. Later I found them on the couch, and my friend said "This cat really feels nice to touch". Her face and Tony's could be best described as "content". Of course the cat had a very special extremely loud purr just for her.

So, the conclusions drawn from my very subjective experiment is that our pets really enrich our lives. It would be safe to speculate that, yes pets reduce stress levels in their owners. If you have a pet yourself, you probably agree!

Try your own experiment.... Ask your friends and coworkers about their pets and soak up the good feelings they radiate. Enjoy.

# Apologies, Forgiveness and Empathy

We live in a world where when someone wrongs us, often we are told "I'm sorry" and the reply is usually "never mind", "forget about it" or "it's nothing". This works 99.9% of the time. But what about when someone has hurts us intentionally - obviously premeditated and/or repeated over a long period of time?

When things like this happen, well-meaning people tell us that we have to forgive in order to heal. This often leaves the "victim" wondering if there is something wrong with them because they can't "forgive".

Warning, the following is a bit disturbing - but has a happy ending.

John and Jane Anyman live in a neighborhood house with their 2 children Jim and Susie. Their next door neighbors Cathy and Steve Goodneighbor have 2 children, Sarah, Charlie and a playful and friendly puppy named Rufus. John is known in the neighborhood as a very nice guy. The two families get together often.

Rufus has a bad habit of digging under the fence, getting out of the yard and chasing moving vehicles. The Goodneighbor family works very hard to keep Rufus inside.

One day Rufus gets out and chases John who is riding his bike. John is very annoyed at the dog and tells Jane that "something will have to be done about THAT dog. People shouldn't be allowed to have dogs like that." His tone of voice is very odd and frightens Jane.

Time goes by…Rufus gets out and chases John again. John, who has been carrying a stick, brutally hits the dog over the head. At dinner, he brags to Jane, Jim and Susie how he "took care of the obnoxious dog".

Later, the Goodneighbor children found Rufus beaten and dead. They were traumatized and very sad. Another neighbor had seen John beat Rufus. He told the Goodneighbors. Steve tells John that someone beat Rufus to death and asks him "Did you see anyone hit the dog?"

John has several choices here. He can:

1.  Deny any knowledge.
2.  Blame the Goodneighbors for "making him do it". Say "Sorry, but you should have kept the dog inside – he was a menace to everyone."
3.  Admit and Apologize. Say he was terribly sorry to have acted so cruelly. Say that he didn't mean to cause the Goodneighbors so much pain and grief. Ask if there is anything that he can do to help them feel better (and do it!).

Let's consider the possible outcomes for each of John's choices above...

1.  Denial:
    The Goodneighbors, John's family and the rest of the neighborhood know that he did it. They are likely to conclude that he is a cruel, abusive person.
2.  Blaming the Victims:
    The Goodneighbors will probably feel angry at John's statement that they "made him" do it. Again, they are likely to conclude that he is a cruel, abusive person - who feels entitled and justified in his abuse (no remorse).
3.  Accepting Full Responsibility:
    The Goodneighbors would feel he is remorseful. In time, they may begin to believe John's act was a mistake instead of deliberate malice. If he follows through with restitution, they may be able to re-connect fully.

The Happy Ending:
Before Jim, Susie Goodneighbor was married to a verbally and emotionally abusive man. She knew from her Abuse Survivor's Group literature that John's cruelty to animals was a big RED Flag of a potentially abusive person. She talked to Jane who confirmed that John sometimes was verbally hostile and when drinking tended to get into fist fights. The two ladies convinced John to seek counseling.

The Anyman's are a happier family now. The neighborhood once again views John as a good guy who made a cruel mistake rather than someone to avoid.

AND... John recently bought a puppy for the Goodneighbors AND one for his own children!

Most of us, at one point in our lives, find ourselves struggling to either apologize for a serious wrong or struggling to forgive one. If you find yourself in this position and looking for answers, the following may help:

Forgiveness Is NOT:

1. Forgetting – if you were wounded enough to require forgiveness, you may always have a memory of it.
2. Excusing or condoning - the wrong should not be denied, minimized, or justified.
3. Reconciling – forgiving does not necessarily mean reestablishing the relationship.
4. Weakness – forgiving does not make you oblivious to cruelty.

A Sincere and Complete Apology IS:
Quick after event - minimize suffering.

1. Specific - "I am sorry I did X, Y, Z".
2. Empathetic - "I am sorry X,Y,Z hurt/embarrassed/humiliated etc. you".
3. Regretful (asks for forgiveness) - "I truly regret that I caused you pain/trouble/money, etc. Please forgive me."
4. Sincere - "How can I make it up to you?" Or "I will change my behavior to avoid this again".
5. Restorative - Follow through with promises made.

This even works for something as simple as being late for a meeting. Instead of saying "sorry", try "I am sorry for being late and wasting your time. Next time I will leave home earlier. May I buy you a cup or coffee to make it up to you?" See how that makes the recipient feel like you care? That you empathize ...

Both forgiveness and sincere apologies require EMPATHY. Empathy is what makes us able to connect... to truly love one another!

# New Year's Resolutions?  Ask for Help

What kind of New Year's resolutions did you make this year?  Did they involve improving your health, fitness, nutrition or related health habits? Every year, many of us start off with good intentions, only to find that "life" gets in the way. A couple of months along we find we are no closer to achieving what we started out to do.

It's easy to justify or excuse these "failures" in a variety of ways.  Maybe it wasn't a high enough priority or we are just too busy and so forth.  But there's one element in all of this that might be overlooked – genuine support and understanding by the people we care about.  An important part of this relationship dynamic is that we feel the person or people closest to us have faith in our abilities to do what we set out to do.

Fitness trainers see this sort of thing a lot.  A person comes for training, gets going well and then starts missing sessions.  When the person is asked why, the answer is usually something like "I feel that I am taking too much time away from my family" or "My wife feels that we are not spending enough time together".  I once had a spouse of a client tell me right in front of the client that the client has started to get fit many times and failed and that now he doesn't believe she can do it!"  I felt the client's hurt and self-doubt with that comment.  Certainly, the comment does not encourage her success.  That's really tough.

If you are having trouble keeping fitness resolutions (or any resolutions) year after year, take a look at your family and friends.  Do you feel that they are enthusiastically supporting your efforts and believe in your ability to accomplish what you start? If not, try to think of some ways to change this situation for the better. Here are some ideas:

Recruit a support group of people who can support and mentor you to help offset some of the difficulties and self doubt you are experiencing.  Your supporters don't have to be fitness enthusiasts (although your trainer is a good place to start).

They can be friends or colleagues whom you enjoy. Even better: talk to people who are accomplishing goals while experiencing resistance or lack of support by their loved ones.

Communicate, communicate, communicate and communicate again!

It's up to you to find a way to communicate the importance of your goals to your family and friends emphasizing your need for them to support you.

Tell your loved ones how difficult this change is for you and how past failures affect your self confidence in this area....and that you need them to help you!

Ask for their suggestions on how you can meet their needs and also accomplish what you want to do.

Try to find out how they feel about what you are doing - if there are fears or insecurities involved. Sometimes there can be hidden agendas, such as a spouse's fear that you getting fit will cause you to change in a negative way or a child who thinks you will spend less time with them. Then, discuss ways to make sure everyone feels secure and happy with any changes in routines etc.

You will be amazed at how much cooperation and enthusiastic support you will receive, just by asking...

# Truth:  Dads are Sexy

Ok guys out there, it's unofficially official.  Hollywood is right.  Involved and caring Fathers are major "Babe Magnets".  How do I know this?  Through observation and experimentation, of course!  A bit of background first.

This is my second marriage and I have a child from the first.  My first husband believed in traditional roles in family life. After we had a child, he left the parenting to me. This was good in many respects, but was very lonely.  Especially as my male friends and work colleagues were highly involved parents and devoted to their families.  I often spent time socializing at family events without my spouse. He was busy working, exercising and socializing with other like - minded people. Although this was not THE reason we divorced, it was a major problem for me in our marriage.  I worried a lot about the effect of the lack of my ex's involvement on my child's emotional well-being.

Through this experience…I grew to admire a great deal the Fathers that I knew who had developed deep relationships with their kids.  It's not easy. Kids are, well…kids.

Sometime after my ex and I split, I met my current husband Dave.  After we had known one another for a few months, Dave said that when I felt like it, he wanted to start getting to know my child.   You see, he has kids from a previous marriage that he is dedicated to.  He told me that he knew that my child and I were a "package deal" and he wanted to grow a relationship with both of us.  Now guys… THAT is sexy to a single mother, believe me. I will leave to your imagination what happened next!

Getting back to the "experiment" and proof of the Babe Magnet Theory… The next time you are at a family gathering where there are Dads with their kids, watch the women.  They are most likely looking at the Dads (not just their own spouse), with a facial expression that seems to be a combination of admiration and…something else.

The women talk about it, too. Usually they say things like, "Look at John, what a NICE man he is!" Another woman will say, "Yea, and a wonderful Dad". That's were my experiment starts. I follow with something like, "That Dad thing is really sexy don't you think?"

After a pause in the conversation and few giggles, inevitably the comments are "yea, it really IS sexy. He's so strong and yet so patient and gentle with his kids", and so forth.

After many conversations like this, I feel that I am beginning to understand what the "something else" facial expression in the previous paragraph is. It's simple: Women ADORE men who genuinely care about, and are there for their kids!

My theory as to why has yet to be tested, but here it is. You see, gentlemen, we modern women are competent, educated, financially independent etc. Yet we still yearn for the knight in shining armor. The classic concept of knight in shining armor in this modern era is obsolete.

The one area in our lives where many of us competent, educated women feel unsure at times is parenting. It's a scary thing! We talk about it constantly. Are we doing the job well, badly, etc..? Lots of advice and experiential knowledge is always passed around. For a man to share the daily parenting and emotionally support the Mom in her role – well, I am guessing that there's not a Mother out there reading who would disagree that these men are the knights in shining armor of our time – our heroes!

The world is a better place because of you – the involved and caring Dad. All of you are heroes…and heroes are Babe Magnets.

…A toast to the great Babe Magnets of the world: past, present and future!

# Achieving Your Goals — Words Make a Difference

Kids have the most amazing insight if you stop and listen to them. Our daughter has an adult relative who lives far away who said to her "I wish I could see you more often". Do you know what she said later? I don't think he means it, or he would see me more often. Good observation.

Let's look at this more closely. When the relative above says "I wish", this person is indicating that 1) they have not made a decision to make it happen and 2) the ability to make visits more often is not within his/her power. To that, I say poppycock!

The decision to "make it so" is the key. Not the how, or why. For any goal, one just has to decide to it and then figure out how. The how will follow. To achieve a goal, it's crucial to decide to do it. It doesn't matter really how or whether you feel that circumstances are outside your control. The means to accomplish this goal will present themselves after you decide. Waiting to think about it or wish about it moves one no closer to achievement. .. and wastes time that could be used constructively toward the goal.

Ok, ok, Nike beat me to it....

To get what we want, we need to get rid of the words "would", "could", "should", "wish", "might" and replace them with "I will" or "I won't". There's no doubt that the Nike slogan has appeal: Just Do It!

If you look at the cause and effect decision making that we do for so many of our decisions, it's very simple: deciding to do it should be first, then how. How many times have you dwelled on making a decision because you started thinking about the how and got stuck? I have, a lot. Unless I take notice, this is the first place I go. It has kept me from taking positive actions more than once.

Many people are comfortable in their world of would, could and should. It's easier to make excuses for failure that way. No promises made to anyone (including oneself), just wishful thinking. Of course, like our daughter pointed out, it's almost always a failure mindset. Without commitment there is no action.

An easy example of this that we all can relate to is diet and exercise. Many of my friends wish they weighed less or "had a body like X". Deciding to get fit and eat right is the first step. The how becomes evident with a bit of studying and organization. Next thing you know… a whole new fit body!

So, it's more the wisdom of our grandfathers and grandmothers than modern science.

It goes like this.

1. Consider decision and its impact to you and your important people
2. Decide to do it or not
3. Then, figure out how

I am working on replacing the "would, could, should" in my vocabulary with "I will, I can, I shall and you bet!". I have been amazed at the difference that one simple paradigm shift has made in my life. Just Do It!

# Seeking Purpose vs. Happiness

Shmuley Boteach, an accomplished theologian, writer and moral leader, writes in his article "Six Values for Raising Outstanding Children" that it is important to stress purpose as opposed to happiness. He goes on to say that telling kids, "I just want you to be happy" is one of the silliest parenting mantras ever. What if being a lazy beachcomber, womanizer or drug dealer makes him happy?

Really makes you think doesn't it?

Boteach's premise is that it is the pursuit of PURPOSE rather than pursuit of happiness that makes people happiest. If we devote ourselves to a purpose that we find meaningful, fulfillment and happiness will follow. Let's work through that idea....

How often in your life have you heard people say "I deserve to be happy", "Life is too short..." etc? But why do we feel like we are simply entitled to be happy? Are we expecting others to do it for us? How? And is our own happiness the only reason that we exist? Big questions!

If you are among us "over 40" crowd, no doubt you have experienced some sort of "mid-life crisis" that is the brunt of so much humor. Doesn't the very core of a mid-life crisis lie in seeking meaningfulness in our lives?

If the thinking is that happiness alone is the reason we live - any changes brought on by the mid-life crisis will not bring us to the answer to the "why am I here" question.

Personally, when I went through a mid-life crisis brought on by divorce, my first thought was what will I do now to make myself happy? This line of thinking was also taken by my ex who wanted a divorce because "he deserved to be happy". It's a common line of thinking.

But when I hit the bottom of my emotional low, I started taking stock of things in my life that gave me happiness. The "aha!" moment came with the realization that I was really happy doing things to contribute to the lives of others:

raising my child, my job lecturing at a university and teaching fitness classes. I became very thankful to have so many opportunities and skills to give to others. It was these things that gave me a sense of feeling valuable, which got me out of bed every morning and through those tough times.

Now, when I meet someone else going through a difficult life transition, I listen for comments like "I have to keep going for my kids" or "my parents need me". These comments show that although the person has it tough, they will get through it all ok. They have purpose; a reason to persevere.

And of course, it's really a lot about perception of the worthiness of your individual pursuits is it not? If you are happy with your life, my guess is that probably because you feel you are a contributing member of society - that what you do is important. It may not be that your job is socially valuable (although most jobs are in some way). But you live your life in a way that gives value to someone else, be it your kids, your spouse, your parents or... the world.

Assigning meaning to your life right now is a matter of bringing the sense of purpose to down to a day to day level. Ask yourself: what is the real motivation for doing the things you do?

Why do you go to work? What contributions do you make in your job to enrich the lives of others? Some jobs are easy to place value. If you work as a fireman, a stay-at-home parent or garbage collector, these jobs make direct contributions to society. If you work as an accountant or office administrator though you may have to look a bit deeper. Let's not discount that working to contribute money to the family is valuable.

What do you do to take care of yourself and why? Exercise, eating right, relaxing and getting medical checks are some ways to take care of yourself. Do you take care of yourself so you look good or because your family, friends and neighbors value you? For most of us it's a complex combination of these things.

If you do volunteer work or contribute to charity, why? Why do you spend time with your family members? What do you do with them? What do you do to enrich their lives? What is your contribution to your friendships?

If you look closely, you will find that the most meaningful things in your life involve giving your unique gifts to others in some way. Real joy comes from giving.

So, it comes down to this: humanity. It's by giving to others that we make ourselves happy. Visualize how you want to be remembered at the end of your life, and you will find the answer to the "why am I here" question. Do you want to be remembered as a great Father, Mother, Citizen, Philanthropist, Friend, Worker...?

Make the world a better place.... live with purpose. Live with joy.

# The Science of Lust and Love

Lust? Love? Is there a difference?

Thinking back to the last time you were newly in love, it will come as no surprise to you that the chemicals released into the blood when you were in the attraction stage are very different than those released later in the relationship. After all, if you had stayed in that new love stage, you wouldn't be unable to accomplish anything except to spend your days pining away for your lover.

Scientists are beginning to identify not only the chemicals involved with "being in love" but also the parts of the brain that are activated. It seems to be an explanation for the anecdotal seven year itch. Well, actually it's anywhere from 4 to 7, depending on the scientist or journal you are reading.

According to researchers, lust, is the sensation that causes us to go out looking for a mate. It's the chemicals estrogen and testosterone that are at work here.

Then there's attraction or being "love struck" . This is the part where you lose your appetite, can't sleep, get sweaty palms and higher heart rate etc. This keeps us going back for more of this person. The love chemicals at this stage are mostly the same ones that are increased whenever we have a new adventure or excitement: the monoamines. These include dopamine, norepinephidrine, phenylethylamine (PEA) and serotonin. Basically, these affect us as if taking amphetamines, stimulants and painkillers!

Dopamine makes us feel happy while serotonin and norepinephidrine make us feel more excited. PEA is the big player here which excites us and helps the transition from lust to love. It's this chemical rush caused by PEA that creates the addiction to being in love we here so much about (Isn't there a song title of the same name?).

Some people jump from relationship to relationship just for the high of the in love feeling. No doubt, the in love chemicals are HARD and addictive drugs.

Alas, after a couple of years of the excitement stage comes the attachment stage. These processes overlap one another in that the in-love chemicals don't just disappear but lessen over time and are replaced with other chemicals.

At this stage, oxytocin, the same chemical involved in childbirth and bonding to the infant, shows up in the blood of both men and women . This stage is often referred to as the attachment stage. Oxytocin is released during orgasm in both men and women. It has been postulated that the more sex the couple has, the more bonded they will become. That's a good tick by nature, don't you think?

Vasopressin, also called the monogamy hormone, comes into play during the attachment phase as well. Vasopressin seems to keep us protective of our mates.

Other chemicals, called endorphins, are released during and after sex. These give us that "feel good feeling" similar to the feeling after a hard exercise session (endorphins are also released during exercise).

An observation: the in-love chemicals take about 2 to 3 years to fade out and be replaced by the bonding chemicals. Have you noticed that this is the time when many people start to find their mates not as interesting or exciting as they once did? Has this happened to you? The person hasn't changed. The chemicals that attracted you to them have faded. Many people, however, find that the attachment feel good chemicals are much more fulfilling than the attraction chemicals.

Pheromones are the smell chemicals that signal sexual attraction or repulsion. No matter how much you like someone, if they do not smell good to you, the sexual attraction just doesn't work. It's said that women on birth control pills will subconsciously seek out men who smell like good protectors and fathers —because the pill simulates pregnancy. But sometimes when these women go off the pill, they suddenly find their mate doesn't smell attractive anymore. Bummer!

In conclusion: the attraction chemicals fade at about 2 to 3 years and are replaced by the bonding chemicals. The bonding chemicals actually interfere with the exciting "in-love" chemicals and create a more "comfortable" bonding love which lasts another few years.

Evolutionarily, the theory is that the couple stays together long enough to raise a child out of infancy. Then both men and women (yes, women are not built for monogamy either) move on and repeat the process. It's good for the gene pool.

So, if you are addicted to the love/lust chemical high, it's very important to keep your sexual and romantic life exciting and new. How to do that? Well, that's a good question for a relationship/marriage counselor!

# The Myth of the Work Life Balance

Isn't balancing work and life tough? I mean really! Even if you feel like you have the greatest balanced life possible – sometimes it just gets to be too much. You know what I mean?

Let's break this down: there are 24 hours in a day. 7 days in a week. That's 168 hours per week. We sleep 8 hours per day. So that's 56 hours per week. That gives us 112 useable hours in the week.

Out of those 112 hours: (note much of this is "guessimation" for illustration purposes only)

Eating: 2 hours per day
Driving in car: 1 hour per day
Exercise: 1 hour per day
Personal Hygiene: 30 minutes per day
Children's attention/homework: 2 hours per day
Cleaning Up Home and Work: 1 hour per day
Connecting to friends: 30 minutes per day
Work: 8 hours per day
16 busy hours per day or 112 hours per week. Hey, it's balanced…NOT!

That's because, it's very rare to have an exacting day like the above. There's doctor's appointments, extra time at work, shopping, meal preparation/acquisition, traffic jams, etc. The list can and does go on and on.

Of course, we need time to "ourselves", time for our spouses, special time for each child individually, time for our parents, time for our friends and just time to relax. How?

Diverting from my usual style of offering solutions, I am going to stick my neck out and say….to me, the work life balance has become a myth.

Someone suggested to me a while back a way of thinking about this: break down activities into: "the things I love to do", "the things I have to do to get what I want" and "the things I have to do to maintain myself (sleep, etc)".

What is being suggested here? It's that maybe the key is not so much to find a better way of managing time – it's to find a better way of perceiving the way it is already being managed. An attitude change so to speak.

Here's an example (my day):

**"Things I Love to Do":**

- Most work tasks

- Help child with homework

- Spend time with my family

- Exercise

- Connect with friends

- Putting my child to bed

- Eat

- Sleep

**"Things I Have to Do to Get What I Want":**

- Drive in the Car

- Clean up home and work (This one is a struggle!)

- Help child with routine tasks (I want a healthy, happy, well adjusted child)

- Some work tasks

**"Things I have to Do to Maintain Myself":**

- Showering

- Food preparation

When I started looking at it from this perspective, it occurred to me how great my daily life is. Most of things I do daily fall into the "Thing I Love" category. The majority of the work I do is great, the majority of the time I spend with my child is great, and I love to eat and sleep! Do I still miss on many things I feel that I should be doing? Of course! But looking at it from this perspective gives me a daily sense of gratitude for the structure of my life as it is now, today. It also helps avoid the "I should have done more for me" feeling.

On the tough days, those days when I have to do more of the "things I have to do to get what I want" it's easy to do them because not everyday is like that and I know that if it became so, I would make appropriate changes to do more of the "things I love to do" everyday.

Feeling overworked and under-appreciated? Sometimes all it takes is a change in perspective. To quote one of my favorite singers: "It's not getting what you want, it's wanting what you got"!

# RESOURCES

**Isn't Vegan a Planet in the Next Solar System?**
1. High Protein Diets: Separating Fact from Fiction by Stephen Byrnes www. mercola.com.
2. Listing of amino acid composition of proteins: www.csmngt.com/amino_acids.htm.

**To Stretch or Not to Stretch...**
Derrick and Webb, Sports Injuries: Diagnosis and Management
www.brighamandwomens.org. Women and Yoga..

**Is Body Awareness an Undergarment?**
Franklin, Eric "Discovering Muscular Imbalances" Human Kinetics Inc.
www.usapowerlifting.com/committees/sportsmedicine/hartle03.shtml
www.shapeshiftermagazine.com/6/02.htm

**Not All Carbohydrates are Created Equal**
1. www.healthyeatingclub.com/info/articles/diseases/glycaemic-index.htm
2. www.drweil.com/u/QA/QA326589/h
3. www.drmirkin.com/nutrition/9566.html
4. www.mendosa.com/gilists.htm

**Too Much of a Good Thing?**
The American College of Sports Medicine, "Overtraining with Resistance Exercise," www.acsm.org.

**Natural is not the Same as Organic**
Organically grown foods: Evaluate your options. www. MayoClinic.com

**Are We Having Fun Yet?**
1. "Holistic Health News, Remedies for Anxiety" http://www.holistic-online.com/remedies/anxiety/anx_exercise.htm
2. "Managing Stress with Regular Exercise", http://www.dukemednews.org/news/article.php?id=8484

**Combating the Effects of a Desk Job**
"The Weak Point Workout" by Scott Hudson. http://www.mensfitness.com/fitness/100

**Have a Six Pack**
Spencer Pilates Instructor Certification Manual

**Health Habit Sabotage**
"Habits that Hurt Your Health". www.shape.com

**The Bigger, the Better?**
"For Portion Control, Look to the Container"
http://www.cnn.com/2006/HEALTH/07/30/diet.cues.ap/index.html

**The United Colors of....Fruits and Vegetables!**

1. "What is ORAC? How Foods Can Help You Fight Cancer". By Susan Dixon http://www.cancer.med.umich.edu/learn/nutorac.htm#list
2. "ORAC Values of Fruits and Vegetables" http://www.drdavidwilliams.com/nc/ORAC_values.asp

**Is It Just a Mid Life Crisis?**
1. http://www.menstuff.org/issues/byissue/andropause.html
2. http://www.andropause.com
3. http://www.midlife-passages.com/hormone.htm
4. http://www.andropausecanada.com/when.php

**Are Exercising to Burn Fat and Exercising to Burn Calories the Same Thing?**
1. Energy Systems in Sport & Exercise, http://www.sport-fitness-advisor.com/energysystems.html
2. Metabolizing Fat and Carbohydrate ,By Jason R. Karp, M.S. http://www.fitnessmanagement.com
3. Understanding how energy is supplied for activity helps make sense of exercise and diet regimens.
By Donna J. Terbizan, Ph.D., FACSM, and Brett A. Dolezal, Ph.D.
4. http://www.fitnessmanagement.com

**The Vitamin D Debates Continue**
1. The Vitamin D Newsletter 08/20/05. John Cannell
2. http://www.thaifoodandtravel.com/features/vitaminD.html
3. The Micronutrient Information Center, Linus Pauling Institute, Oregon State University.
4. http://lpi.oregonstate.edu/infocenter/vitamins/vitaminD/index.html
5. The Mayo Clinic Newsletter, Drugs and Supplements Section. http://www.mayoclinic.com/health/vitamin-d/NS_patient-vitamind
6. "The Miracle of Vitamin D" by Krispin Sullivan CN. http://www.westona-price.org/basicnutrition/vitamindmiracle.html

**Are You Fit...Emotionally?**
http://www.ediets.com/news/article.cfm/cmi_2422447/cid_7

**Type D Personality?**
1. Type D Personality: The Impact of Stress and Loneliness on Our Health, by Robert Brooks PhD.
2. http://www.drrobertbrooks.com/writings/articles/0605.html
3. Harvard Health Publications http://www.health.harvard.edu/press_releases/type_d_personality.htm

**Wellness and Making Good Choices**
http://www.answers.com/topic/wellness

Neuro-Linguistic Programming for Fitness?

1.http://www.nlpmind.com/nlp.htm

2.http://www.nlpschedule.com/w_neuro_linguistic_programming_definition.
html

## Words Do Hurt – Stop Bullying from Affecting Your Health

1.    Bully Busting By Marti Olsen Laney, Psy.D.

2.    http://www.selfgrowth.com/articles/Laney1.html

3.    Pity, Not Love. By:Hara Estroff Marano

4.    http://psychologytoday.com/articles/pto-20040726-000008.html

5.    I'm Rubber and You're Glue: Handling Emotional Bullies By: Edel Jarboe

6.    http://www.pioneerthinking.com/ej_rubber.html

7.    Workplace Bullying. By Martin Maylor

8.    http://ezinearticles.com/?Workplace-Bullying&id=445916

9.    Evans, Patricia. The Verbally Abusive Relationship. Adams Media, 1996.

10.    Evans, Patricia. Controlling People.  Adams Media,2002.

## Fit Body Equals Fit Brain

"Working out is good for body and brain" by Mary Carmichael.

## The Longevity Diet?

http://www.calorierestriction.org.

## Pets and Stress

1.Cardiovascular Reactivity and the Presence of Pets, Friends, and Spouses: The
Truth About Cats and Dogs.Karen Allen, PhD, Jim Blascovich, PhD and Wendy
B. Mendes, MS

2.http://www.psychosomaticmedicine.org/cgi/content/abstract/64/5/727

## Lifestyles, Behaviors and Lower Risk of Death

Mayo Foundation for Medical Education and Research (MFMER)

## Is it Perfume or Poison?

1.    Neurotoxins: At Home and the Workplace, (Report by the Committee on
Science & Technology, U.S.House of Representatives, Sept.16, 1986. (Report
99-827)

2.    "Living Healthy in a Toxic World," David Steinman 1996

3.    "Stink-Free Office Mates," Natural Health Magazine, Nov./Dec. 2000.

4.    http://www.ourlittleplace.com/chemicals.html "How Fressh is the Air
Freshener?"

5.    http://www.time.com/time/health/article/0,8599,1664954,00.html?cnn=yes

## The Focusing Illusion

1.    Staying happier for longer.  By Professor Martin Seligman.

http://news.bbc.co.uk/1/hi/programmes/happiness_formula/4903464.stm

2. Study Shows "Grass is Greener" View Usually False http://www.mercola.com/1998/archive/grass_is_greener.htm

**How to Use Criticism as a Learning Tool**

1. The Achievement Paradox, 2002, by Ronald A. Warren. Library. www.newworldlibrary.com

3. http://theroadtoceo.com/How_to_React_to_Criticism.html

4. http://zenhabits.net/2007/09/how-to-accept-criticism-with-grace-and-appreciation/

**Green Cleaning Ideas for Your Home**

http://en.wikipedia.org/wiki/Hygiene_hypothesis

**Let's Compromise...Aerobic vs Anaerobic Training**

1. "Aerobic vs Anaerobic, What's the Controversy About?" Eddie Lomax.

2. http://www.boeafitness.com/articles/exerciseandweighttraining/2006_01_10_4010.php

3. International Fitness Professionals Association, "Personal Fitness Training Manual".

**The Science of Lust and Love**

1. 'The Chemistry of Love" by Dr. Susan Block http://www.counterpunch.org/block02122005.html

2. "The Science of Love – Cupid's Chemistry" by Claire McLoughlin
http://www.thenakedscientists.com/HTML/articles/article/clairemcloughlincolumn1.htm/

**Exercise for Physical, Emotional and Intellectual Fitness**

http://www.usnews.com/blogs/on-fitness/2008/4/17/how-exercise-revs-up-your-brain.html

**Is Bottled Water Really Better?**

API Press Release: "Bottled water has contaminants too, study finds" By Jeff Donn.

**Is It Just a Mid Life Crisis?**

1. http://www.menstuff.org/issues/byissue/andropause.html

2. http://www.andropause.com

3. http://www.midlife-passages.com/hormone.htm

4. http://www.andropausecanada.com/when.php

**It's Not Just What You Eat, Its How You Cook It**

1. Press release April 24, 2007, Mount Sinai Medical Center.

2. Grilled, Fried, or Broiled Meat Produce Toxins Called Advanced Glycation End Products (AGEs)

3. http://www.discount-vitamins-herbs.net/n-607-glycation-carnosine.htm

**The Many Disguises of Mono Sodium Glutamate**
1.   Everything You Need To Know About Glutamate And Monosodium Glutamate http://www.ific.org/publications/brochures/msgbroch.cfm
2.   Interview with Dr. Russell Blaylock on devastating health effects of MSG, aspartame and excitotoxins http://www.newstarget.com/020550.html

**Wellness and Making Good Choices**
http://www.answers.com/topic/wellness

**Sugar Feeds Cancer?**
1.   "The Good Fight". Health Sciences Institute
2.   http://www.hsibaltimore.com/ealerts/ea200407/ea20040701.html
3.   "Sugar Link to Small Bowel Cancer". PersonalMDhttp://www.personalmd.com/news/a1997030601.shtml"Cancer Decisions Newsletter" http://www.cancerdecisions.com/082102_page.html"Study Suggests Possible Link Between
4.   High Starch Diet and Pacreatic Cancer".Science Dailyhttp://www.sciencedaily.com/releases/2002/09/020904073950.htm


**Slim People at Risk for Fat Related Health Problems?**
1.   Subcutaneous and Visceral Adipose Tissue: Their Relation to the Metabolic Syndrome Bernardo Léo Wajchenberg http://edrv.endojournals.org/cgi/content/full/21/6/697
2.   Abdominal fat and health riskshttp://www.diabetesselfmanagement.com/article.cfm?aid=930
3.   Strength Training in Diabetes Managementhttp://www.redorbit.comUltrasound measurements of intraabdominal fat estimate the metabolic syndrome better than do measurements of waist circumerence1,2 Ronald P Stolk, Rudy Meijer, Willem PTM Mali, Diederick E Grobbee and Yolanda van der Graaf on behalf of the Secondary Manifestations of Arterial Disease (SMART) Study Group http://www.ajcn.org/cgi/content/full/77/4/857